LONG TERM CARE
TEST-TAKING REVIEW
FOR NURSE AIDES
& ASSISTANTS

D1373329

LONG TERM CARE

TEST-TAKING REVIEW FOR NURSE AIDES & ASSISTANTS

SKILLS, DRILLS, and PRACTICE TESTS

Prepare for Certification

BARBARA A. VITALE, R.N., M.A.
Huntington, New York

PATRICIA NUGENT, R.N., Ed.D.
Huntington, New York

THE C. V. MOSBY COMPANY
St. Louis • Baltimore • Philadelphia • Toronto   1990

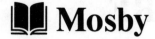

Printed in the United States of America

The C. V. Mosby Company
11830 Westline Industrial Drive, St. Louis, Missouri 63146

ISBN 0-8016-5221

TP/P/P 9 8 7 6 5 4 3 2 1

Dedicated to
Joseph M. Vitale ▪ Neil J. Nugent
for their love and support

Preface

The nurse aide's unique role in long term care has never been more challenging. In most instances it is the nurse aide who (1) identifies that the condition of a resident has changed and notifies the nurse for professional assessment, (2) provides for activities of daily living, (3) provides emotional support, and (4) may even play the role of family. Nurse aides in long term care are usually caring, hard working, over-worked, and undervalued.

The American public has finally recognized the important role of nurs aides in the provision of dignified, quality care to elderly and infirmed people residing in nursing homes across the United States. With the predicted increase in the percent-age of elderly in our society as baby boomers age, there will be a need for better educated and increased numbers of entry-level care givers in long term care. With the passage of The Omnibus Reconciliation Act of 1987 (OBRA), nurse aides must pass federally mandated, state issued nurse aide training and competency evalua-tion programs by January 1, 1990, to be registered and able to work as nurse aides in long term care.

The setting of minimum standards of education and practice for the nurse aide-level care giver glows with the promise of improved care at the bedside. OBRA, while necessary and desirable, has placed a particular strain on presently employed nurse aides because they must pass their state's nurse aide testing program to keep their jobs. Over 625,000 presently working nurse aides must prepare for and take and pass competency evaluation programs to work as nurse aides in long term care. OBRA uses the title *nurse aide* in relation to the bedside care giver. However, in the long term care industry the title *nurse assistant* is used interchangeably with nurse aide depending on the state or facility. To avoid constantly referring to nurse aide/nurse assistant, the initials NA will be used for these titles throughout the book.

Few books are on the shelves to assist this level of care giver to prepare for state competency examinations. This book is designed for presently working nurse aides and nurse aide students who are preparing to take a competency test to be registered to work in long term care. It can also be used by nurse aide educators for assess-ment, learning, and evaluation purposes. This book focuses on:

- Anxiety reducing techniques that can be used to control anxiety producing situa-tions and responses
- Study skills that will help to increase knowledge and the retention of information

- The problem-solving process and how this problem solving approach can be used to organize and provide care
- Test-taking skills to develop logical thinking when reading and answering test questions
- Practice questions with the reasons for the correct and wrong answers, to increase knowledge about nurse aide practice
- Test drills, with the reasons for the correct and wrong answers, to increase knowledge about nurse aide practice
- Test drills, with the reasons for the correct and wrong answers, to simulate state competency examinations

In writing this book we want to acknowledge those nurse aides who are devoted to the residents for whom they provide care. All too often nurse aides receive little recognition or gratitude for their service. We would like to thank the facilities and nurse aides who participated in the field testing of questions. We are also grateful to Tom Manning, President of the Manning Company, for recognizing the educational needs of nurse aides and to Jeanne Toma, our editor, who worked with Tom Manning to facilitate the prompt delivery of this manuscript to the public. Most importantly, we would like to thank our husbands and children for their love and support: Joe, Joseph, John, and Christopher Vitale and Neil, Kelly, and Heather Nugent.

How to Use This Book

There are four important concepts about learning.
- Learning occurs best when there is a readiness to learn.
- The learner must be motivated.
- Learning takes place within the learner.
- The learner must be an active participant in the learning process.

The fact that you bought this book shows that you are ready and motivated to learn. You have a goal: to pass your state nurse aide competency test. This book was written to help you achieve that goal. As you use this book you will recognize that you are expected to be an active participant in your own learning. Remember, learning takes place within the learner, and the benefits you receive will depend on the extent of your effort.

The content of this book was designed to be used in a planned way to maximize effective study and learning. Chapter 5, Practice Tests for State Nurse Aide Evaluation Programs, contains three practice test drills. Before you begin studying this book, take one of the three test drills in Chapter 5 as a pre-test to get a sense of your level of nurse aide knowledge and test-taking ability. After you complete studying Chapters 1 through 4, take another one of the test drills. After you complete the practice questions and answers in Chapter 6, take the last of the three test drills as a post-test. The order in which you take the tests does not matter. The purpose of these tests is to simulate nurse aide competency tests, demonstrate growth, and motivate. If you are studying effectively, your test scores should improve from test to test. These practice tests were specifically placed in Chapter 5 so that you would not accidently take them all at one time if they appeared in Chapter 1.

The chapter topics progress in a specific order from Chapter 1 through Chapter 4 and should be studied in this order. Chapter 1, Controlling Anxiety, provides techniques that will help you to reduce your anxiety so that it does not interfere with learning. Chapter 2, Study Skills, presents specific and general study skills that should improve the learning and retention of information. Chapter 3, The Problem-Solving Process, discusses how a problem solving process is applied to nurse aide practice. Chapter 4, Test-Taking Skills, presents specific and general test-taking skills that should improve your ability to answer multiple choice questions. When you have completed Chapter 4, remember to take the second test in Chapter 5.

Chapter 6, Practice Questions with Reasons for Answers, contains practice test questions grouped within content areas. The reasons for the correct and wrong answers are included for each question. The purpose of this chapter is to provide you with an opportunity to practice answering test items. In addition, the reasons for the answers help you to learn or review the common principles of nurse aide practice. To be most useful, it is suggested that you answer the questions within a content area after having studied this information in your nurse aide testbook. When you have completed Chapter 6, remember to take the final test in Chapter 5.

The Omnibus Reconciliation Act of 1987 (OBRA) uses the title *nurse aide* in relation to the bedside care giver. However, in the long term care industry the title *nurse assistant* is used interchangeably with nurse aide depending on the state or facility. To avoid constantly referring to nurse aide/nurse assistant, the initials NA will be used for these titles throughout the book.

Successful preparation for a nurse aide competency test requires a huge effort on your part. Hopefully, this book will make that task easier. Good luck on your state competency test.

Contents

CHAPTER 1

Controlling Anxiety

Anxiety is felt by most people at some point in their lives. It is an uneasy feeling of the mind and body caused by inner feelings, thoughts, desires, actions, and drives related to a threat. Anxiety is based on emotion, not logic. For most people, important examinations are emotional, stressful experiences. You may have physical symptoms when you feel threatened or in danger. This is the body's way of protecting itself from harm. As your anxiety increases, it can prevent you from remembering facts or details and from doing your best work. If tests make you anxious and nervous, you need to learn how to limit your emotional responses and think logically. With practice, YOU CAN BE SUCCESSFUL at limiting your anxious responses.

Before you can control test anxiety, you have to understand what it is that threatens you and how you react to that threat. Concerns are negative and bad if they cause physical and emotional responses that interfere with your ability to feel calm and in control while studying or actually taking a test. However, concerns about tests are helpful and good when you know what they are and when they motivate you to study harder. There are several concerns that cause test anxiety that are common to most people. These concerns are centered on:

1. How well you are prepared to take the test, or the feeling that you are never quite ready to take the test.
2. How others, such as family members and friends, will feel about you if you do not pass the test.
3. How you will feel about yourself if you do not pass the test, and what it will do to your confidence and self-esteem.
4. How the future may change and how goals may need to be changed if you do not pass the test.

It is important to recognize that each person may have a different concern or combination of concerns that trigger test anxiety. If you can look honestly at what makes you afraid and confront your concern, you may be able to reduce test anxiety.

You can also reduce test anxiety by being overprepared for a test, developing a positive mental attitude, using breathing and muscle relaxation techniques, and exercising regularly. These approaches must be practiced prior to test taking for them to be successful in controlling your anxiety. When you gain control of anxiety-producing situations, you can successfully reduce anxious responses and improve your thinking ability, thereby improving your test performance.

BEATING TEST ANXIETY

Skill 1—Be overprepared for the test

One cause of test anxiety centers on how well you are prepared to take the test. The more prepared you are for the test, the more able you are to challenge the fear of not being prepared. Study your nurse aide textbook. When you think you know the information, keep studying the same information to reinforce your learning. Use this book to practice test-taking, which will enhance your learning and improve your test-taking skills. Overpreparation is the best way to fight the fear of not being prepared. Nothing will build confidence and reduce anxiety more than knowing the subject well.

Skill 2—Develop a positive mental attitude

A cause of test anxiety can center on how you will feel about yourself or how others will feel about you if you fail a test. However, your value as a person should not be linked with how well you do on a test. Your self-worth and your test performance are separate things. If you were raised thinking that you were good when you passed a test and bad when you failed, then you must change your thinking. You may also be concerned with how your life and goals may have to change in the future if you do not pass the test. Thoughts about the future can be realistic, but when they are negative they can be defeating. Negative thoughts must be turned into positive thoughts to reduce anxiety and build confidence.

Before you can learn new skills to reduce test anxiety, you have to be willing to face your concerns. Anxiety is usually a feeling related to an unknown threat; for example, not knowing the outcome of a test. When negative thoughts enter your mind, write them down. Examine these thoughts and try to pinpoint your concerns. Identify what is most frightening to you. Once you know what worries you the most, you have identified your enemy. You are ready to begin turning negative thinking into positive thinking.

When you think negatively about yourself or your performance, these negative statements may cause you to be less alert and reduce your concentration. If you think you may fail, you may fulfill your prediction. Therefore, the most important part in successful studying and test-taking is a POSITIVE MENTAL ATTITUDE. When you say things like, ''I'll never pass this test, it's too hard,'' ''I can't do it,'' or ''I'm so stupid,'' then you are getting lost in negative and failing statements. STOP IT IMMEDIATELY! Challenge negative statements every time they come into your mind. For example, if you say, ''I'm never going to be able to pass this test,'' challenge this negative statement with: ''Never is a stupid word''; ''I am over-reacting''; ''If I study hard, I know I can pass.'' Challenge negative statements because they may cause you to give up before you begin, even though you have a lot of knowledge.

A positive mental attitude can also be developed by thinking of happy endings. For example, imagine how you will feel when you are notified that you have passed. Think of the relief that you will feel when your goal is achieved, and the pride you will feel in your achievement.

To change negative thinking into positive thinking is not easy because the old habits and ways of thinking that developed over time must now be unlearned. You may say, "These challenging techniques are silly games. I cannot see myself doing them." Although these activities may seem like games, they give you control over your attitude. They keep your thinking positive and constructive rather than negative and destructive. Be assured, they work in reducing anxiety. If you need to develop a positive mental attitude, then you owe it to yourself to give these techniques a chance so that you can better use your abilities. You can develop an **"I can do it"** attitude.

Skill 3—Perform breathing exercises

It is a known fact that people react physically to a fear or threat. You breathe faster and more shallowly in response to stress. A good way to manage feelings of anxiety is by being aware of your breathing pattern and using breathing techniques to cope with stress. The Lamaze method of childbirth uses controlled breathing techniques to reduce pain. Controlled breathing can also be effective during an examination when there is high anxiety, such as at the start of the test, when facing a difficult question, or when there is only a short time left to complete the examination. These critical times are when you can use controlled breathing. Take a slow deep breath and then let it out smoothly and slowly. Every few minutes you can repeat these steps. Be careful not to take deep, rapid breaths. Wait a minute or two between breaths or you will hyperventilate and bring on a dizzy feeling. Breathing exercises work to reduce anxiety because breathing is something you can control.

Skill 4—Promote muscle relaxation

Muscle relaxation is the tensing and relaxing of each muscle group of your body until all parts of your body are relaxed. This is an excellent way to reduce the muscle tension associated with anxiety. If you can interrupt the tension cycle related to anxiety, you will probably increase your test performance. Muscle relaxation is a skill that must be learned and practiced. Find a quiet place and sit in a comfortable chair. Take a deep breath and let it out slowly, close your eyes, and you are ready to begin. Tense and then relax each muscle group in your body. Tense a muscle for ten seconds. Feel the sense of tension in your muscles. Then relax that muscle for ten seconds. Feel the sense of relaxation in your muscles. Tense and relax muscles in a smooth manner. Do not rush or move quickly. If the muscles still feel tense after you have tensed and relaxed an area, then repeat tensing and relaxing the same area. Tense and relax each muscle group starting with your toes and working upward to your head. Move through the following list of muscle groups, tensing and relaxing several times.

- Bend your toes forward—RELAX
- Stretch your toes upward—RELAX
- Bend your ankles forward—RELAX
- Bend your ankles backward—RELAX
- Rotate your ankles—RELAX
- Press your thighs and calves to the chair—RELAX
- Squeeze your buttocks together tightly—RELAX
- Arch your back and pull back your shoulders—RELAX
- Pull in your abdomen and round your shoulders—RELAX
- Hang your arms and lift your shoulders up toward your ears—RELAX

- Make fists, bend your elbows, and tense the biceps (The biceps are the ones that are tensed when children say, ''Feel my muscles.'')—RELAX
- Bend your head forward toward your chin—RELAX
- Bend your head backward by looking at the ceiling—RELAX
- Bend your head to the right side and try to touch your ear to the shoulder—RELAX
- Bend your head to the left side and try to touch your ear to the shoulder—RELAX
- Roll your head around your shoulders—RELAX

The face:

- Raise your eyebrows—RELAX
- Open your mouth wide—RELAX
- Drop your chin with your mouth open—RELAX
- Make a big smile—RELAX
- Press your lips tight together—RELAX
- Pucker your lips as if you were going to kiss someone—RELAX
- Squeeze your eyes shut—RELAX

Now try to concentrate on how relaxed you feel. If the tension cycle has been broken, you should feel like a balloon that has lost its air. You may even feel like you are floating. Practice these techniques every day. When you feel tense during a test, you can call on these techniques, which will have become second nature to you. They work best when you have practiced because you have programed an automatic relaxation response to your actions.

Skill 5—Perform regular exercise

Regular exercise helps you use and get rid of nervous energy. Exercise, such as jogging, fast walking, aerobic exercise, swimming, and bicycle riding, three times a week for 20 minutes is a great way to stay physically fit and mentally calm. Your exercise should be well planned. Start within your ability level. Remember, you are not preparing for the Olympics. Do not run a mile when you have never done it before. You could hurt yourself and actually lower your resistance to stress. Start slowly and with short distances. Gently increase your speed and distance as you naturally improve. Fitness and feeling well are your goals. You will find that this type of program will help you to stay calm in tense situations.

CONTROLLING ANXIETY IMMEDIATELY BEFORE AND DURING A TEST

If you have been exercising and practicing your relaxation and breathing techniques, challenging negative statements, and you are overprepared, then your anxiety should be tolerable and under control. However, at the last minute, such as immediately before or during a test, you may feel anxious. To reduce this anxiety you must regain control. When you control your activities, belongings, personal space, physical responses, and attitudes, you will create a sense of calm and reduce anxiety. Some of these techniques are reinforced in Chapter 4, Test-Taking Skills. However, they are discussed here because they are done specifically to reduce anxiety.

CONTROLLING ANXIETY BEFORE THE TEST
Skill 6—Control your travel

When you know the location of the test site, make a dry run to find out how long it takes to get there. Travel at the same time of day you will be traveling on the day of the test. If it is far from where you live, you might stay at a nearby hotel to reduce travel time or anxiety about being late because of heavy traffic. Pamper yourself; you deserve it. This may be money well spent because it will help to support your self-worth and a sense of calm.

Skill 7—Control your daily routine

Maintain a normal routine the day before the test. Do not stay up late, eat normally, and do not drink more than one beverage or drink with caffeine. Caffeine can overstimulate and affect attention and concentration.

Skill 8—Control your study habits

Do not study by cramming the night before the test. Cramming only clutters and confuses the mind, which can make you more anxious. Have confidence in what you already know and maintain a positive mental attitude.

Skill 9—Control the preparation of your test-taking tools

Make a checklist of things to bring with you, such as your favorite chewing gum, a good luck medal, sharpened pencils, or a pen. Add to this list any identification forms or admission cards that may be required by the rules of your state. Reread the state test instructions a week before the test so that you do not forget anything important that you may have to bring to the test.

CONTROLLING ANXIETY DURING A TEST
Skill 10—Control your environment

Arrive early so that you can have the choice of any chair. If you find radiators too hot or windows too drafty, avoid these areas. Choose a seat away from the doors and the proctor's desk. These areas can become noisy and disrupt your sense of calm. You have the ability to control part of your testing environment.

Skill 11—Control your physical and emotional preparation

Do some last minute breathing and relaxation exercises just before the test. Remind yourself how well prepared you are and how much you know. Maintain a positive mental attitude.

Skill 12—Control your physical responses

During the test if you feel tense, your breathing becomes shallow and rapid, or you find that your mind goes blank, STOP! Take a deep breath and let it out slowly. Do a quick miniversion of your breathing and relaxation exercises and then go back to the test. Your daily practice of breathing and relaxation exercises should have prepared your body to respond by calming down. Once again you should feel in control.

Skill 13—Control your attitude

If you get a negative thought, STOP! Challenge the negative thought. Replace the negative thought with a positive thought and then go back to the test. Control your thoughts and maintain a positive mental attitude.

CHAPTER 2

Study Skills

Like test-taking skills, the ability to learn effectively is not something you are born with; it is a skill you learn either from a teacher or from your own past experiences. Much of what you learn is from day-to-day living, on-the-job training, or trial and error. However, if you use study skills when you are learning something new, you can probably cover more information, understand more of what you have studied, and remember the information for a longer period of time.

This chapter presents both specific study skills and general study skills. The general study skills include actions that can help you become a successful learner regardless of the topic being studied. The specific study skills section is divided into four sections: knowledge, comprehension, application, and analysis. Each section explains a type of thinking ability and then presents multiple choice questions that are related to each type of thinking ability. Finally, in each section, specific study skills are discussed that may help you increase your ability to use your thinking abilities and learn new information.

SPECIFIC STUDY SKILLS

Types of questions that test thinking ability

Generally there are four types of thinking processes that are tested by multiple choice questions: knowledge, comprehension, application, and analysis. The difficulty of an item will depend upon the type of thinking required to answer the question. Knowledge questions are usually the easiest questions to answer because all you have to do is memorize facts, while analysis questions are the hardest questions to answer because you have to know and understand a lot of information to answer the question.

In the examples throughout this section, the asterisk (*) is in front of the correct answer.

Knowledge questions

Knowledge questions are those that test your ability to recall facts or information. To answer these questions you need to memorize information. For example, these questions might ask you to remember normal values for vital signs, define a word, or select a step in a procedure.

_____ **EXAMPLE 1**

What is a normal rectal temperature?
   (A) 95.0 F
   (B) 97.6 F
  *(C) 99.6 F
   (D) 101 F

To answer this question you had to know the normal range for a rectal temperature.

_____ **EXAMPLE 2**

NPO means a person:
   (A) Should just drink clear fluids.
  *(B) Can have nothing by mouth.
   (C) Is on complete bed rest.
   (D) Has a low salt diet.

To answer this question you had to know the meaning of the abbreviation NPO.

_____ **EXAMPLE 3**

What should the nurse aide do *first* before getting the equipment for a procedure?
   (A) Position the resident for the procedure.
   (B) Pull the curtain around the bed.
   (C) Raise the bed to its highest position.
  *(D) Tell the resident what is going to be done.

To answer this question you had to know the beginning steps of any procedure.

Specific study skill 1—Memorization

Questions that expect you to recall facts require you to have a certain body of knowledge. At first information can be learned by memorization. Repeating facts over and over (saying them within your mind, speaking them out loud, or writing them on paper) uses repetition as a way of getting yourself to remember facts. This type of learning can be carried a step further by making a set of flash cards. Take blank index cards and write a different fact on each card. Carry the cards with you during the day and when you have a few minutes test yourself with the flash cards. This reinforces learning because it is spread over time and it uses repetition. Facts learned by simple repetition use short term memory and are usually quickly forgotten. However, they can be remembered longer if additional study skills are used or the information is often applied.

Specific study skill 2—Acronyms

Memorized facts can be remembered better if the fact is connected to a word where each letter of the word has meaning. These words are called **acronyms** and are used to jolt the memory. For example: **AIDS** stands for **A**cquired **I**mmune **D**eficiency Syndrome; when assessing for pain, **PANIC** stands for **P**eriod of time, **A**rea affected, **N**onverbal actions, **I**ntensity of pain, and **C**haracter of pain. Be creative and make up your own words that have meaning for you in relation to content you are trying to remember. It does not matter if it is not a regular word, as long as the word has meaning for you.

Specific study skill 3—Alphabet cues

Memorized facts can be remembered better if the fact is connected to letters of the alphabet. This skill can be used to trigger the recall of related information. For example: the **ABCs** of cardiopulmonary resuscitation are **A**irway, **B**reathing, and **C**irculation; when assessing for urinary retention remember the **4Ds**—**D**ribbling, **D**iscomfort, **D**uration, and **D**istention. You can use any combination of letters. They do not have to follow the alphabet in order. The combination of letters just needs to have meaning for you.

Specific study skill 4—Acrostics

Memorized facts can be remembered better if the fact is connected to a phrase, motto, or verse where the first letter of each word is a key to open the door to a mental thought. These phrases are called **acrostics** and are used to recall information. For example, **E**veryone **N**eeds **T**ender **L**oving **C**are is a phrase that can be related to the principles of proper communication.

Everyone has the right to tender loving care
Nonjudgmental attitude promotes communication
Tell only health team members about the communication
Listening is necessary to get the message
Center your reply on the resident

Specific study skill 5—Repetition

Sometimes information is learned because of day in and day out use of the information. For example, if you take 15 to 20 rectal temperatures a day it does not take long to learn that the normal rectal temperature ranges between 98.6 and 100.6 F. Sometimes information is learned through repeated actions. Using information or putting theory into practice helps you to remember it better.

Comprehension questions

Comprehension questions are those that test your ability to understand information. To answer these questions you need to know the meaning of the information you have memorized. For example, these questions might ask you to explain something, measure an amount of fluid, or predict an outcome.

_____ **EXAMPLE 1**

Why do elderly people most often become incontinent of urine?
  *(A) Their bladder muscles become weak.
  (B) They do not drink enough fluid.
  (C) Their diets lack fiber.
  (D) They want to control others.

To answer this question you not only needed to know that the elderly become incontinent, but you had to understand why they become incontinent.

_____ **EXAMPLE 2**

If a person on intake and output drinks 12 ounces of milk, the nurse aide should mark on the resident's record an intake of:
  (A) 36 cc (ml).
  (B) 90 cc (ml).
  (C) 240 cc (ml).
  *(D) 360 cc (ml).

To answer this question you not only needed to know that one ounce is equal to 30 cc (ml), but you had to multiply 12 ounces by 30 cc (ml) to get the correct answer.

_____ **EXAMPLE 3**

A person who drinks large amounts of fluid will:
  (A) Have dark colored urine.
  (B) Overwork the kidneys.
  *(C) Have to urinate more often.
  (D) Stretch the bladder too much.

To answer this question you not only needed to know that the fluid a person takes in is related to urinary elimination, but that the more a person drinks the more often the person will urinate.

Specific study skill 6—Understand the information

Memorized information is usually remembered if it is understood. Try to determine how the information relates to a resident situation. Attempt to put the information into a context that has meaning. When you learn a piece of information, ask yourself "why" or "how" this information is important. The reason why something happens or how an action meets a resident's needs will help you to better understand information. For example, you may know that an elderly person can become incontinent. In addition to memorizing this information, you should ask, "Why do elderly people become incontinent?" The answer to this question can be obtained from the nurse, a nurse aide book, or a book about the aging process. There is a reason for everything that happens and for everything you do.

Specific study skill 7—Study in small groups

First you should memorize information and study why or how the information is important. Once you have studied by yourself, then meet with another person or a small group of persons studying the same topic. Some people might say, "Misery likes company." Sharing a stressful situation, such as the need to take a test, may reduce anxiety. While this is a positive outcome, it is not the main purpose of small group work. Working with others gives you a chance to:

Listen to the thoughts and ideas of others

Share your thoughts and ideas with others

Evaluate each other's thinking, understanding, or facts

Help someone understand information you know

Learn information someone else knows

Reinforce or firm up your understanding of information

Debate or discuss the information being learned

Specific study skill 8—Practice skills

Comprehension questions test your ability to understand information. A question that asks you to measure intake and output requires that you know that 30 cc (ml) equals one ounce. It also measures your understanding of how many ounces are involved and multiplying the number of ounces by 30 to get the correct answer. You must understand simple multiplication and how to compute or calculate a problem. Once you know how to measure ounces and multiply numbers, then you can practice problems. You can practice by making up resident situations and then calculating the results. You can also practice by keeping a daily intake and output record on yourself or family members. For example, each time you have something to drink, calculate how many cubic centimeters (cc), or milliliters (ml) you had. Computing numbers is a skill that uses the understanding of mathematics. Skills are learned, improved, and perfected by practice.

Application questions

Application questions are those that test your ability to use information. To answer these questions you need to take information you know and understand and apply that information in a situation. The question usually starts with a short story or description of a resident situation. Then you might be asked to plan an activity, provide care, or respond to a resident. When faced with a question that asks you to use information, you must use problem solving skills. You need to look at the question and identify key words (collect data), analyze what is really being asked (analyze data), review the four possible answers (explore choices), and make a decision (intervention). The answer chosen should be based on the understanding of a basic concept, a scientific principle, and/or logical thinking.

_____ **EXAMPLE 1**

When a resident cannot always control his urine, what should he be encouraged to do?

    (A) Stay in his room.
  *(B) Urinate every two hours.
    (C) Limit his fluid intake.
    (D) Wear disposable diapers.

To answer this question you needed to know that the elderly are sometimes incontinent due to weakness of the muscles used to control urination. You also had to know that urinating every two hours may help them to regain control of their bladder.

_____ **EXAMPLE 2**

When a resident with a urinary tube (Foley catheter) is transferred to a wheelchair, the drainage bag should be:

    (A) Placed in the resident's lap.
    (B) Hung from the handgrips of the wheelchair.
  *(C) Hooked on the wheelchair below bladder level.
    (D) Put on the floor under the wheelchair.

To answer this question you needed to know that a urine collection bag should be kept lower than the bladder to allow urine to drain by gravity. You also had to know that hooking the bag on the side of the wheelchair would permit urine flow by gravity.

_____ **EXAMPLE 3**

A resident who was incontinent of urine says to the nurse assistant, "How can you stand this, it is such a messy job." What is the best thing the nurse aide could say?

  *(A) "This must be hard for you."
    (B) "I am used to it by now."
    (C) "It is part of my job."
    (D) "It's better than a bowel movement."

To answer this question you needed to know that people who are incontinent feel out of control and are upset. You also had to know that accepting and focusing on these feelings helps them to feel better.

Specific study skill 9—Identify commonalities

Studying for application questions begins with memorizing and understanding information. You cannot apply information in a new situation unless you understand the basic concepts involved. When you study basic concepts, such as a wide base of support being necessary for balance or preventing falls, ask yourself how this information could be used in different resident situations. For example, a wide base of support being necessary for balance would apply to:

Keeping your feet apart when moving a resident up in bed

Widening the legs of a mechanical lift before it is moved

Using a walker or cane

This study skill is very useful when working in a small group. Review a basic concept and then brainstorm the different ways the information can be applied in resident situations.

Specific study skill 10—Identify reasons for actions

Application questions are based on scientific principles or basic concepts. There should be a reason for everything you do for a resident. Every time you do something for a resident, ask yourself, "What is the reason for this action in this situation?" For example, giving a back rub to a resident who cannot move increases circulation to the area, which will prevent bedsores. However, giving a back rub to a tense, anxious resident may help to reduce muscle tension and promote relaxation. Another example would be that giving a bed bath to a resident who is incontinent cleans the skin. However, giving a bed bath to a resident with a fever helps to reduce the temperature. In each situation the care given was the same, but the reason for the care was different. Understanding why you do things in similar or different situations will help you to understand and apply basic principles in new situations.

Analysis questions

Analysis questions are those that test your ability to understand and use different kinds of information. To answer these questions you need to take several pieces of information that you know and understand and use that information to answer the question. For example, these questions might ask you to come to conclusions, identify differences, or interpret information.

_____ EXAMPLE 1

If the amount of fluid a person drinks is less than normal, the person's urine will look:

   (A) Cloudy.
   (B) Straw colored.
  *(C) Dark yellow.
   (D) Pink tinged.

To answer this question you needed to know the color of normal urine and that cloudy urine and pink-tinged urine are abnormal. Finally, to pick the correct answer, you had to know that when persons drink a small amount of fluid, their urine will be dark yellow (concentrated).

_____ **EXAMPLE 2**

The resident with the highest chance of getting a bedsore is the person:
- (A) Walking around.
- *(B) On bed rest.
- (C) Allowed out of bed.
- (D) Using a wheelchair.

To answer this question you needed to know that pressure causes bedsores and people on bed rest tend to lie in one position. To pick the correct answer, you also had to know that people who are out of bed or use a wheelchair have less pressure against the skin than those on bed rest.

_____ **EXAMPLE 3**

Which of the following vital signs should be immediately reported to the nurse?
- (A) A pulse rate that is 80 and regular
- (B) A rectal temperature of 99.6 F
- (C) A blood pressure reading of 120/80 mm Hg
- *(D) A respiratory rate of 36 per minute

To answer this question you needed to know all the normal values for temperature, pulse, respiration, and blood pressure. To pick the correct answer, you had to identify which option was outside the normal range.

Specific study skill 11—Identify differences

Questions that expect you to analyze the information are the most difficult because you must be able to use several facts that you have memorized and understand. They are like application questions, but instead of using one piece of information, analysis questions require you to handle a lot of information at one time. For example, to be able to identify an abnormal vital sign from among a group of different vital sign results, you need to know the normal range for each of the vital signs and understand what would be abnormal results for each. Another example would be, that if you are asked to identify the person who has the highest chance of getting a bedsore from among several people, you would have to know what a bedsore is, what causes a bedsore, and what specific situations relate to the causes of bedsores. To prepare for these type of questions, you have to first memorize and understand information and be able to apply it in a simple situation. Once you understand a body of information, then you can try to connect or interrelate the information to similar or different situations. After you have memorized and understand the normal values for vital signs, then identify vital sign results that would be abnormal. You could even go a step further and explore why a vital sign might be abnormal. For example, an elevated pulse could be caused by anxiety, activity, or a fever. When studying bedsores you learn that they are caused by pressure. Try to identify resident situations that would cause pressure on the skin and then try to identify resident situations that would not cause pressure on the skin. This study skill helps you to review the commonalities (what is similar) and differences (what is not similar) in information.

Specific study skill 12—Practice test-taking

Since practice makes perfect, it is a good idea to practice taking tests. Although this study skill is discussed under analysis questions, it should be used to prepare for knowledge, comprehension, and application questions as well. Answering practice questions and reviewing the reasons for the correct and wrong answers should help you to:

Learn new facts

Understand information

Apply information you know and understand

Reinforce what you know and understand

Become comfortable with answering multiple choice questions

Use and perfect test-taking skills

Manage your time during a test

Increase your confidence

Reduce your anxiety

GENERAL STUDY SKILLS

General study skill 1—Set a regular time to study

Set aside time to study. It takes practice to learn any skill. Spending time reading a book, memorizing facts, or practicing taking tests is the same as practicing serving a tennis ball. The more you do it, the better you get at performing the skill. The study schedule must be reasonable and workable. Figure out what is realistic for you. Study for about one hour and then take a break. Long periods of study can be tiring, and you will not learn as much as when you study and are rested. Generally, one- to three-hour study periods with a ten-minute break each hour are effective. Studying an hour every day is less tiring and more efficient than studying seven hours in one day.

General study skill 2—Study in a quiet comfortable environment

Find a quiet place to study where you will not be distracted by family members or phone calls. Do not study with the television or radio on. Noise or interruptions can decrease your ability to concentrate. Select a comfortable table and chair. Because you will be taking the test at a desk or in a chair with an arm table, avoid studying in an easy chair or couch. Ensure that you have good light. Try to simulate the environment in which you will be taking the test.

General study skill 3—Gather your tools

When preparing to study, collect all your tools, such as your textbook, a dictionary, your class notes, extra paper, a highlighting pen, and several pens or pencils. All necessary equipment should be gathered before you start. This will prevent interruptions later.

General study skill 4—Compare class notes to the textbook

When reading the textbook, highlight important words or concepts with a highlighting pen. Keep highlighting to a reasonable amount. Do not highlight entire paragraphs. This defeats the purpose of highlighting. You want to be able to look at a page and pick out the most important content. Review your class notes and identify the important information. Now, compare your class notes with the same information in the textbook. Information is sometimes better understood when it is learned from a variety of viewpoints. Also, the repetition may increase your ability to remember the material.

General study skill 5—Restate content in your own words

Read a section of your class notes or your textbook. Look up a word you do not know in an English dictionary. If the word is a medical term, look it up in a medical dictionary. Then, try to put the material into your own words. When you learn information in the context of your own vocabulary, the chance that you will understand and remember the information will probably increase.

General study skill 6—Use spare time efficiently

Most of your studying should be done during your regularly scheduled study periods. However, during the day everyone has periods of time that are not productive, such as when waiting for an appointment or commuting on a bus. When this happens to you, use the time to study. Carry flash cards, a list of vocabulary words, or the steps in a procedure so that you can learn new information or review learned material when you have unexpected time.

General study skill 7—Seek help

The principles of nurse aide practice are not always easy. The content uses medical vocabulary, and the concepts can be complex. Only you know if you do not understand certain information. Have the courage to admit your limitations and seek immediate help. Sometimes another person, such as the instructor or a classmate, can be helpful. If the other person is a classmate, make sure that person is a reliable source of correct information.

CHAPTER 3

The Problem-Solving Process

The nursing process is a scientific problem-solving process used by nurses to identify resident needs and organize and deliver nursing care. However, the concept of problem solving is not unique to nursing. All people can use problem solving to meet the daily demands of their jobs. Problem solving consists of a series of steps that can be followed to identify and solve problems within the level of their job descriptions.

The nurse aide (NA) performs simple and basic resident care under the direct supervision of the nurse. However, there are many times the NA can use problem-solving skills to organize and deliver assigned care. Of course, when the problem-solving process is used by the NA, it must be used at the NA's level of practice. The NA's level of practice includes basic procedures related to resident needs, such as safety, emotional and physical comfort, personal hygiene, nutrition, elimination, and exercise. The NA is also responsible for making simple observations of the resident.

NAs should understand the problem-solving process because it provides a framework or blueprint that can be followed when giving assigned care to residents. Because this process is helpful to providing care for residents, test questions on NA examinations will reflect the steps of the problem-solving process. NAs should refer to the steps in this process when answering test questions in class or when taking their state test for registration. Understanding the problem-solving process will help to identify what the question is asking.

This chapter reviews each of the four steps in the problem-solving process: **assessment**, **planning**, **implementation**, and **evaluation**. Sample test questions based on each step of the problem-solving process are presented. Finally, how the problem-solving process is used in answering the questions is discussed.

ASSESSMENT

Assessment, the first step in the problem-solving process, has three parts. First, you must collect information about a resident. Second, you need to analyze information to decide if it is normal or abnormal. Third, you need to respond to abnormal signs and symptoms. Your actions within these steps must be within the role of NA practice.

Collecting information

You can gather information from different sources, such as from the resident, family members, or medical records. Medical records that you can use might include weight books, positioning sheets, and the NA assigned care flow sheet (accountability record). Information that you collect from the resident can be objective or subjective. **Objective** information is gathered through the use of the senses of seeing, hearing, smelling, and touching. Examples of objective information might include crying behavior, a measured blood pressure, a foul odor to stool, or cold, clammy skin. **Subjective** information includes feelings that must be described by the resident. Examples of subjective information might include a resident's complaint of dizziness, pain, fear, or sadness.

When collecting information about a resident, objective information can support subjective information. For example, a resident states that he is very sad. This is subjective information because the resident tells you about his feelings. You observe that the resident is crying and has a poor appetite. These are examples of objective information because they are behaviors that you can see. The crying and lack of eating are objective information that supports the subjective information, which is the resident's expression of sadness.

Analyzing information

Analysis, the second part of assessment, is the hardest part of assessment. It is difficult because it requires you to come to a conclusion about the information collected. To come to a conclusion about whether information is important or not requires you to understand the principles of NA practice. You need to know about how the normal body works, what are the common reactions to the stress of illness, and what signs and symptoms are abnormal.

Responding to collected information

The last part of assessment is related to how you respond to the information collected. If the information is within normal ranges and/or is expected behavior, it does not need to be immediately reported. However, if the information collected is outside the normal range or is important to the health and safety of the resident, then it should be immediately reported to the nurse. When responding to resident needs, you must know the role of the NA, which includes both the NA's responsibilities and limitations. In other words, you should know what you can do and what you cannot do when responding to information. If you know when information is normal or abnormal, the limitations of your practice, and when to report to the nurse, you should provide safe care to residents during the assessment phase of the problem-solving process.

Questions that measure the nurse aide's ability to make assessments

Test questions can measure your ability to assess a resident's condition within the NA's level of practice. This is done by asking you to collect information, identify normal or abnormal signs and symptoms, or correctly respond to collected information. Questions that ask you to respond to collected information are the hardest because you have to look at the information, determine its importance, and choose the answer that is the correct action in response to the information. The following are examples of questions that test your ability to collect information, analyze the importance of information, and respond correctly to assessments within the role of NA practice.

In the examples throughout this chapter, the asterisk (*) is in front of the correct answer.

_____ **EXAMPLE 1**

Besides a blood pressure machine (sphygmomanometer), what piece of equipment would the NA need to take a person's blood pressure?
- (A) Thermometer
- (B) Wheelchair
- (C) Watch
- *(D) Stethoscope

This question tests your ability to identify equipment that is used to collect vital signs. To answer the question correctly, you have to know that a stethoscope and blood pressure machine (sphygmomanometer) are needed to measure a blood pressure. You can also correctly answer the question if you know that a thermometer, wheelchair, and watch are not needed to measure a blood pressure. Knowing how to collect information about a resident is part of assessment.

_____ **EXAMPLE 2**

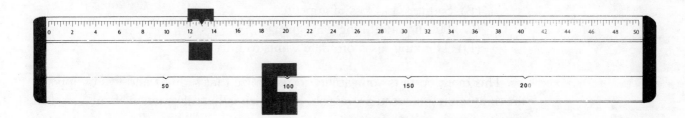

Mrs. Rogers is being weighed on a balance scale. Using the picture above, what weight should the NA record?
- (A) 100 pounds
- (B) 112.5 pounds
- *(C) 113 pounds
- (D) 163 pounds

This question tests your ability to measure the weight of a resident. To answer this question you have to know how to read a balance scale. Collecting important information about a resident is part of assessment.

_____ **EXAMPLE 3**

What is a normal rectal temperature?
   (A) 95° F
   (B) 97.6° F
  *(C) 99.6° F
   (D) 101° F

This is a simple question that tests whether or not you can recognize a value that would be within the normal range for a rectal temperature. To answer this question correctly, you have to know the normal range for a rectal temperature. Answers A, B, and D are all outside the normal range for a rectal temperature. Therefore, answer C is the correct answer. Analyzing collected information is part of assessment.

_____ **EXAMPLE 4**

A resident with cancer has pain that prevents him from doing simple tasks for himself. Which of the following behaviors would show that he is depressed?
   (A) Holding the painful area with his hand
  *(B) Sadness and loss of appetite
   (C) Hitting and biting care givers
   (D) Thinking his roommate wants to hurt him

This question tests your ability to recognize that sadness and loss of appetite are common responses to depression. Recognizing that information about a resident is not normal is part of assessment.

_____ **EXAMPLE 5**

Which of the following vital signs should be immediately reported to the nurse?
  *(A) A respiratory rate of 36 per minute
   (B) A pulse rate that is 80 and regular
   (C) A rectal temperature of 99.6 F
   (D) A blood pressure reading of 120/80

This question tests your ability to recognize an abnormal vital sign and know that it must be immediately reported to the nurse. To answer this question correctly, you must know the normal values for temperature, pulse, respirations, and blood pressure. Then you must know which of the answers is outside those normal ranges.

_____ **EXAMPLE 6**

The NA checks on Mrs. Green and finds her in bed with her eyes closed. Which of the following conclusions should be made by the NA?

    (A) She is feeling withdrawn.
    (B) The resident is sleeping.
  *(C) More information is needed.
    (D) Mrs. Green is unconscious.

This question tests your ability to respond correctly to collected information. This question requires you to analyze whether or not you have enough information to come to a conclusion about the condition of the resident. The NA needs to know the signs, symptoms, and behaviors that support a conclusion. In this question there is not enough information presented in the stem (statement presenting the problem) to support answers A, B, or D.

PLANNING

Planning is the second step of the problem-solving process. It involves input from all members of the health team before goals and care are identified. As an NA you spend a lot of time with residents. NAs usually know their residents well and often gather important information other team members may not collect. Although the nurse develops the nursing plan of care, you can provide important information at nursing team meetings and health team conferences. For these reasons NAs are valuable members of the health team and should be included in the planning phase of the problem-solving process.

Planning usually takes place before care is given. However, sometimes problems arise and plans may need to be changed while in the process of giving care. If the resident's condition changes, the nurse must be notified because the plan of care may also need to change. Therefore, when giving care you must not blindly follow the NA assignment sheet. The resident's condition must be considered and the nurse notified of any changes in the resident's condition.

Questions that measure the nurse aide's ability to contribute to the planning of care

Test questions can measure your ability to help set goals and plan care to assist residents to achieve goals. A resident situation might be described, and you would be asked to identify the correct resident goal or the care needed to achieve a stated goal appropriate to NA practice. The following are examples of questions that test your ability to help set resident goals or plan care within the role of NA practice.

_____ **EXAMPLE 1**

The NA finds a resident spreading stool on himself, the linens, and the bedrails. The resident goal that would be most appropriately met by the NA would be that the resident will:

   *(A) Be clean and dry.
    (B) Stop spreading stool in the future.
    (C) Call the NA for the bed pan.
    (D) Toilet himself when needed.

This question requires the NA to identify the resident's goal that is within the role of NA practice and then focus on the immediate desired outcome (goal), which is to be clean and dry. Answers B, C, and D are more long range and require teaching/training programs. This question tests your ability to identify a resident goal that is the easiest to reach through care given at the NA's level of practice. Keeping residents clean and well groomed is a major role of the NA.

_____ **EXAMPLE 2**

A resident has a decubitus. Which of the following devices should the nursing team plan to use to protect the resident's skin?

   *(A) Sheepskin
    (B) Cane
    (C) Walker
    (D) Splint

This question tests your knowledge about devices that can be used to protect residents. All of the above devices are helpful to residents. However, only answer A, sheepskin, is related to preventing a decubitus. Answers B and C are related to assisting residents to maintain balance, and answer D prevents contractures. Knowing what to do for a resident requires you to first know **how** and **why** you do certain things. To answer this question you have to know that sheepskin reduces rubbing (friction) and allows air to flow through the tufts of lamb's wool between the skin and bed linen. Knowing how and why certain interventions work enables you to understand the purpose of assigned care.

_____ **EXAMPLE 3**

A resident has a weakness on the right side. When planning to help the resident dress, what should the NA plan to do?

   (A) Encourage her to dress by herself.
 *(B) Put her right sleeve on first.
   (C) Keep her in an open backed gown.
   (D) Put her left sleeve on first.

This question tests cause and effect as related to dressing. If you put clothes on the weak side first, then there will be less stress to the joints and muscles of the weak side. Knowing this principle, the NA plans to put clothes on the weak side first. Understanding the cause and effect of care is necessary to give care that is correct to meet the needs of each resident.

_____ **EXAMPLE 4**

Mrs. Cox is always grouchy and bossy and sometimes hits the NA. When giving her care what should the NA do?

 *(A) Include her in as many decisions as possible.
   (B) Avoid her when she is angry.
   (C) Explain that the staff is only trying to help her.
   (D) Stop her grouchy and abusive behavior.

This question tests knowledge of principles related to how to approach the combative, bossy, or grouchy resident. This type of person is usually fighting for control. The behavior is a response to the uncontrollable and scary things that are happening in the resident's life. Therefore, providing chances to make choices gives her more control, which may reduce her combative behavior.

_____ **EXAMPLE 5**

The NA assignment sheet directs the NA to assist the resident in a tub bath at 10 AM. However, the resident has just returned from physical therapy, is very tired, and refuses the bath. What should the NA do?

   (A) Give the bath anyway.
 *(B) Tell the nurse.
   (C) Give a shower instead.
   (D) Cancel the bath.

This question requires you to recognize that the plan of care is never set in stone but must be changed in response to the needs of the resident. Right now the resident's need for rest is more important than the need to be clean. A plan of care should always be changed in response to the changing condition of the resident. To change the resident's plan of care, the nurse must be notified because changing a plan of care is the legal responsibility of the nurse.

IMPLEMENTATION

Implementation, the third step of the problem-solving process, consists of two parts: carrying out the assigned plan of care and recording the care given. You are responsible for providing care assigned by the nurse. However, the assignment must be within the legal limits of the NA's role. Assignments can be indicated on the NA assignment sheet or given verbally by the nurse. Results can be reported in writing on the NA accountability records or given verbally to the nurse. The method used for reporting depends on the nature of the information being reported and the facility's policies and procedures.

Implementing the nursing care plan

To carry out the assigned care, the NA needs to reassess the resident before giving care and while giving care, know when assistance is needed, and provide care using scientific principles.

Before carrying out assigned care, the NA must reassess the condition of the resident. The condition of the resident can quickly change, which will in turn alter the plan of care. For example, it is planned that Mrs. Como is to ambulate 30 feet in the hall. When the NA goes into the room, the resident is short of breath, holding her chest, and complaining of chest pain. It is clear that this should be immediately reported to the nurse because the plan of care may need to be changed by the nurse. As an NA you must reassess the resident before giving the assigned care. This assessment is done within the NA's level of practice.

You must never blindly follow the planned care on the NA assignment sheet without considering both the resident's and your own needs. For example, the NA assignment sheet may tell you that a resident needs the help of one person to ambulate. However, you believe that two people are needed to provide safe ambulation. This should be discussed with the nurse. It is your responsibility to use good judgment based on safety principles and seek help when needed.

The need for more assistance may be different than the physical help of another person. For example, a situation may arise where you feel you need more information about how to do something. You may need to refer to a policy and procedure book, a nurse, or a resource person such as an in-service instructor for help or direction. Because of the ever changing health care setting and new equipment, you may find that you lack the skills to provide safe care. Asking for immediate assistance when the need arises is using good judgment based on principles of NA practice.

NA care is based on a scientific foundation that includes, but is not limited to, the following principles.

- Care should support residents' individual needs.
- Care should include resident involvement as much as possible in the planning and implementation of their own care.
- Care should be directed at preventing complications.
- Care should be directed at achieving identified goals.
- Care should be directed at maintaining the highest level of resident independence and functioning.
- Care should be delivered in a manner that supports resident safety.
- Care should support comfort and hygiene.
- Care should support the emotional, psychosocial, and spiritual needs of residents.

Reporting and recording care given

The NA is responsible for reporting and recording assigned care that is implemented. **Reporting** is the transfer of information to others through spoken words. Verbal reports may be given to the nurse during a shift when an emergency arises or abnormal signs and symptoms are observed. Verbal reports may also be given at the end of a shift to highlight events that occurred during the shift. **Recording** is the transfer of information in written form. Written records commonly used by the NA include the NA assigned care flow sheet (accountability records), positioning sheets, bowel and bladder training records, intake and output sheets, ambulation schedules, percentage of meal intake, and vital sign grafts.

Questions that measure the nurse aide's ability to implement care

Test questions can measure your ability to implement care within the level of NA practice. Situations are presented to test your ability to reassess residents before giving care, determine the need for assistance, implement care based on scientific principles of NA practice, and appropriately report and record implemented care.

_____ **EXAMPLE 1**

The NA is transferring a resident from a bed to a chair. When the resident moves to a sitting position, what should the NA say to the resident to assess her response to the change in position?

(A) "That was very good."
(B) "Hold on to my shoulders."
*(C) "How do you feel?"
(D) "Let's get ready to stand."

This question tests your ability to apply principles of assessment while actually giving care. Dizziness is a common response when an elderly person moves from a lying to a sitting position. The NA would not transfer a resident until after the body has had a chance to adjust to the sitting position and the dizziness passes. The need to assess residents while giving care is part of implementation, the third step of the problem-solving process.

_____ **EXAMPLE 2**

The NA is assigned to a resident who transfers to a chair with a mechanical lift. It has been a long time since the NA used the mechanical lift. What should the NA do?

*(A) Ask the nurse to show how to use the mechanical lift.
(B) Keep the resident in bed for the day.
(C) Ask another NA to explain how to use it.
(D) Use the mechanical lift and hope that you remember.

This question requires you to decide what to do when faced with a situation that requires you to seek help. Answer B can be immediately eliminated since care givers should never provide care based on the needs of the care giver. Answer D can be eliminated because it would be unsafe to proceed with the hope that you get it right. You must be sure of your actions and not just hope that you remember. Answer C can be eliminated because an NA would never be responsible for teaching or supervising another NA. This is the job of the nurse. Therefore, answer A is the only correct answer. This question tests whether you know how to seek help to provide safe care. Providing safe care is part of the implementation step of the problem-solving process.

_____ **EXAMPLE 3**

The nurse asks the NA to do something that is outside the legal scope of the NA role. What should the NA do **first**?
  (A) Do the task and file a grievance later.
  (B) Call the supervisor immediately.
 *(C) Respectfully refuse to do the task.
  (D) Call the union representative.

This question attempts to test your understanding of what should be done when asked to do something that is outside the scope of NA practice. When implementing care, the NA must know the limits of NA practice and be prepared to refuse to do something that is illegal.

_____ **EXAMPLE 4**

When giving a resident a bed bath the water should be:
  (A) 80° to 90° F.
  (B) 95° to 104° F.
 *(C) 107° to 115° F.
  (D) 120° to 130° F.

This question tests your ability to implement safe care. To provide for resident safety when giving a bed bath, the NA must know that the water should be between 107° and 115° F. If it is hotter it can cause a burn or scalding, and if it is cooler it can cause a chill, reduce body heat, and be uncomfortable for the resident. Understanding the principles that guide NA practice enables the NA to provide or implement safe care.

_____ **EXAMPLE 5**

To provide for the safety of a resident who is restrained in a chair in his room, how should the NA position the resident?

   *(A) Near a call bell
   (B) Differently every three hours
   (C) Next to a roommate
   (D) Close to the door

This question requires you to recognize that residents have a right to be able to call for assistance and to have their needs met in a reasonable time period. Long term care standards and guidelines require that residents' rights be met.

_____ **EXAMPLE 6**

A resident is on a restricted fluid intake. What form is used to record how much water the resident drinks?

   (A) Nurses notes
   (B) NA assignment sheet
   *(C) Intake and output sheet
   (D) Weight sheet

This question tests your ability to identify a commonly used form for recording the intake of fluid. Because reporting and recording are important parts of the implementation step of the nursing process, questions that focus on documentation will most likely be on an NA test.

_____ **EXAMPLE 7**

A resident on bed rest is on a turning and positioning schedule/clock every two hours. When the NA signs a signature/initial to the turning schedule, it means that:

   *(A) The resident was repositioned at that time.
   (B) The resident's skin looks better.
   (C) Range of motion was done to all joints.
   (D) The resident was told to turn over.

This question tests your understanding of the purpose of an accountability record or form used by the NA. Responsibility for one's actions within the scope of NA practice is the reason for documenting and is a basic principle related to implementing care.

EVALUATION

Evaluation, the fourth step in the problem-solving process, measures the resident's response to care given, which must then be reported to the nurse. The nurse then identifies whether or not the resident's goals have been met. Evaluation is important because the resident's response or progress toward a goal will determine if the plan of care will continue or be changed by the nurse. If goals are met, then changes are not necessary. If the resident's response lacks progress, then the plan may need to be changed. For example, the goal is, The resident will have a bowel movement in the morning. The plan includes walking the resident and encouraging fluids and foods high in fiber. The next morning the resident does not have a bowel movement. The care given did not help the resident to reach the goal of a bowel movement. Therefore, the plan of care needs to be changed by the nurse. The goal for another resident is, The resident will walk ten feet. The plan includes assisting the resident to sit on the side of the bed for five minutes and then walk the ten feet. While walking, the resident became very weak and was immediately put back to bed. When this was reported to the nurse, the nurse determined that the goal was not met and the plan should be changed. The goal was changed to, The resident's legs will be stronger. The plan was changed to include strengthening exercises of the legs for two weeks before again setting the former goal of ambulating ten feet.

The step of evaluation requires the NA to collect data about the condition of the resident once care is given and report the results to the nurse.

Questions that measure the nurse aide's ability to evaluate a resident's response to care

Test questions can measure your ability to collect information about a resident's response to care. An evaluation question would describe a resident's response to care, and you might be asked to decide if that response was expected or not expected. Another evaluation question might ask if a resident's goal within the NA level of practice was met or not met. In another question you might be asked if the resident demonstrated progress or lack of progress toward a goal. These types of questions attempt to test your ability to evaluate the results of care you have given within the role of NA practice.

_____ EXAMPLE 1

Which of the following is most important to report to the nurse about a resident who was ambulated?
   (A) Where it took place
   (B) How long it took
   (C) When it took place
   *(D) The response of the resident

This question tests your ability to recognize that to evaluate whether a goal is met, one must first collect information about the resident's response to care given. Answer D is the most important because to determine if the goal was met, one must first assess the resident's response to care given and then compare the two.

_____ **EXAMPLE 2**

The nurse aide provides passive range of motion (ROM) to maintain joint movement. This goal would NOT be met if the resident developed a/an:

    (A) Decubitus

    (B) Rash

  *(C) Contracture

    (D) Infection

This question tests your ability to identify a condition that can occur when ROM is NOT effective. Answer C is the correct answer since a contracture causes a decrease of motion in a joint when ROM is not effective. Answers A and B are not related to lack of ROM and joint movement, but to pressure and lack of skin care. Answer D is related to infection management and not ROM and joint mobility.

_____ **EXAMPLE 3**

A resident weighing 165 pounds is on a reduced calorie diet. The resident's goal is to lose two pounds per week. Which of the following weights would meet the goal?

    (A) 167 pounds

    (B) 165 pounds

    (C) 164 pounds

  *(D) 163 pounds

This question tests your general understanding of the concept of comparing goals with outcomes when evaluating a resident's response to care. To answer this question correctly, you had to figure out the goal weight by subtracting two pounds from the original weight of 165 pounds. The correct answer is D, or 163 pounds.

SUMMARY

The problem solving process is used to organize and deliver safe care to residents. The problem-solving process used by the NA must be within the scope of NA practice and not impose on the legal role of the licensed nurse. Assessment permits you to collect, analyze, and respond to information about a resident. Planning involves input from all members of the health team before goals and care are identified. Implementation is the actual carrying out of the assigned plan of care and the recording of care given. Evaluation is the measurement or observation of the resident's response to care and the reporting of this information to the nurse.

The problem-solving process is a dynamic, active, and continuous process. It really does not have a start or finish but goes around like a circle. Sometimes more than one step may be involved at a time. For example, assessment is always ongoing throughout the problem-solving process because the condition of the resident can change at any time. You should understand how to apply this process to meet residents' needs. Understanding the problem-solving process will also help you to decide what a test question is asking. Knowing what the question is asking will increase your ability to analyze which of the four choices is the correct answer. Understanding the problem-solving process should help you to answer questions correctly and improve your test performance.

CHAPTER 4

Test-Taking Skills

The ability to take tests effectively is not something with which you are born, but a skill that is learned. However, you probably do not practice this skill because you do not take tests every day. Most people do not take tests every day because it is not needed for their jobs and it is not a fun activity. It is the rare person who loves to take a test. Tests are often difficult, raise our anxiety, and are a threat to us personally. Test-taking skills cannot replace good study habits or knowledge about the subject being tested. However, when you do take an important test, if you have practiced test-taking skills, you will probably find the test less difficult, be less anxious, and get a higher score than if you did not practice test-taking skills.

There are two factors you must have to score well on a test: you must know the subject being tested, and you must be test-wise. This chapter is concerned with helping you to become test-wise. Being test-wise involves knowing the general strategies related to taking a test and using the specific strategies of how to analyze a test question to increase the chances of getting the answer correct. Although the focus of this chapter is on test-taking skills, hopefully you will also learn how to improve your ability to understand what you have read and increase the knowledge you have about caring for people.

THE MULTIPLE CHOICE QUESTION

What is a multiple choice question? The whole question is called an **item**. Each multiple choice item has two main parts. The first part is the statement that presents the problem. This is the **stem**. The second part consists of all the possible choices. They are the **answers**. One of these answers is the **correct answer**. The answers that are not the correct answer are the **wrong answers**.

In the examples throughout this chapter, the asterisk (*) is in front of the correct answer.

_____ **EXAMPLE 1**

Which of the following is the correct temperature for bath water? (stem)

    (A) 90° F (wrong answer)
    (B) 98° F (wrong answer)
  *(C) 110° F (correct answer)
    (D) 130° F (wrong answer)

The stem + the answers A, B, C, and D = **a test item**.

_____ EXAMPLE 2

To make a bed that will help prevent bedsores the bottom sheet should be: (stem)

    *(A) Pulled tight. (correct answer)
    (B) Loose at the toes. (wrong answer)
    (C) Changed every day. (wrong answer)
    (D) Mitered at the corners. (wrong answer)

The stem + the answers A, B, C, and D = a test item.

THE STEM

The stem is the statement that presents the problem. It should contain all the information needed to make the item clear and specific. The stem can be written as an incomplete sentence or as a complete sentence that asks a question. The stem can be stated in terms of what should be done (a positive statement) or what should not be done (a negative statement). Some stems may ask a question in relation to a picture, chart, or graph.

When the stem is a complete sentence

When the stem is a complete sentence it will be a statement that asks a question and it will end with a question mark (?).

_____ EXAMPLE 1

Which of the following would have to be measured if the resident was on intake and output?

    (A) Applesauce
    (B) Rice pudding
    (C) Pureed fruits
    *(D) Ice cream

_____ EXAMPLE 2

Which blood pressure is normal in the elderly?

    (A) 90/60 mm Hg
    *(B) 130/84 mm Hg
    (C) 150/96 mm Hg
    (D) 200/110 mm Hg

_____ EXAMPLE 3

Which of the following actions by the nurse aide (NA) would help a resident meet a basic physical need?

    (A) Pulling up the side rail after care
    (B) Encouraging a resident to do an activity
    (C) Answering a call light quickly
    *(D) Placing a resident back in bed to sleep

When the stem is an incomplete sentence

When the stem is an incomplete sentence, it will be only part of a sentence. It becomes a whole sentence by being completed with one of the answers. The answer that is the correct answer is the only one, out of the four possible answers, that will complete the sentence correctly.

_____ **EXAMPLE 1**

When a person's urine output is less than the fluid taken in, the person will:
   *(A) Gain weight.
   (B) Become incontinent.
   (C) Get diarrhea.
   (D) Urinate more often.

_____ **EXAMPLE 2**

A restraint should be tied to the:
   (A) Side rail.
   (B) Headboard.
   *(C) Bed frame.
   (D) Bedside table.

_____ **EXAMPLE 3**

Mr. George has not been sleeping well at night. To help him, the NA should:
   (A) Suggest that he exercise before bedtime.
   (B) Ask the nurse to give him a sleeping medication.
   (C) Give him a warm cup of tea at bedtime.
   *(D) Encourage him to be up and active in the daytime.

When the stem is a positive statement

When the stem is written as a positive statement, the correct answer will be something that is **correctly related** to the statement or something that **should** be done. A positively worded stem tries to find out if you have correct information and know what should be done.

_____ **EXAMPLE 1**

The best way to keep a resident from falling out of bed is by:
   (A) Telling the resident to call for help.
   (B) Putting the bed in the lowest position.
   *(C) Raising both side rails of the bed.
   (D) Placing an overbed table in front of the resident.

_____ **EXAMPLE 2**

After restraints are applied the resident gets agitated and more confused. What should the NA do?

(A) Tell the resident to calm down and relax.
(B) Remove the restraint until the resident calms down.
(C) Isolate the resident in a quiet room.
*(D) Explain to the resident the purpose of the restraint.

_____ **EXAMPLE 3**

What is the main cause of obesity (overweight)?

*(A) An intake of more calories than are burned for energy
(B) A serious mental condition causing overeating
(C) A problem with glands preventing loss of weight
(D) Diabetes which prevents the breakdown of sugar

When the stem is a negative statement

When the stem is written as a negative statement, the correct answer will be something that is **not related** to the statement or something that **should not** be done. A negatively worded stem tries to find out if you know the exception, can tell what should not be done, or can pick out errors. Words in the stem that will clue you to the fact that it is a negative statement are **except**, **not**, or **never**. When a negative word is used it may be brought to your attention by dark type (**except**), italics (*never*), or capitals (NOT).

_____ **EXAMPLE 1**

When applying wrist restraints the NA should do all of the following **except**:

*(A) Use a double knot to secure the straps.
(B) Pad the wrists with something soft.
(C) Tie the straps to the bed frame.
(D) Place a call bell within reach.

_____ **EXAMPLE 2**

When taking a rectal temperature with a glass thermometer, which of the following should *never* be done by the NA?

(A) Turn the resident on the side first.
*(B) Let go of the thermometer when it is in the resident.
(C) Shake down the thermometer before using it.
(D) Report an abnormal temperature to the charge nurse.

_____ EXAMPLE 3

An agitated resident tells the nurse aide that life is no longer worth living and she wants to die. Whom should the NA NOT tell about this statement?

(A) The resident's doctor

(B) The social worker

*(C) The resident's roommate

(D) The charge nurse

When a stem uses a picture

When a stem is a question that refers to a picture, graph, or chart, the correct answer will be influenced by the drawing. For example, you may have to identify a piece of equipment, plan care, or come to a conclusion.

_____ EXAMPLE 1

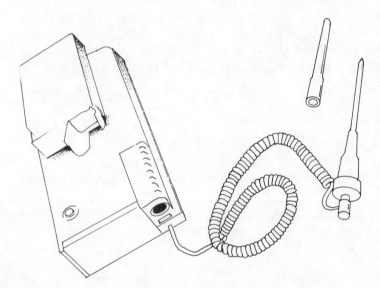

When taking a resident's vital signs, which vital sign can be taken with the piece of equipment shown above?

(A) Pulse rate

*(B) Body temperature

(C) Respiratory rate

(D) Blood pressure

_____ EXAMPLE 2

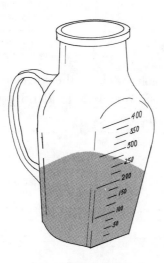

A resident on intake and output (I&O) urinates. According to the urinal above, how many cubic centimeters (cc), or milliliters (ml), should the NA record on the I&O record?

   (A) 175 cc (ml)

*(B) 200 cc (ml)

   (C) 250 cc (ml)

   (D) 300 cc (ml)

_____ **EXAMPLE 3**

DAILY INTAKE AND OUTPUT RECORD

RESIDENT NAME: DATE:

11-7 FLUID INTAKE			11-7 FLUID OUTPUT			COMMENTS
TIME	AMOUNT	TYPE	TIME	AMOUNT	TYPE	
12:00	140	Juice				
1:00	120	water	1:00	320	urine	
5:00	300	coffee	3:00	200	urine	
7:00	300	water	5:00	100	urine	
			6:00	60	Vomitus	
TOTAL:			TOTAL:	680		

A resident is on I&O. According to the I&O record above, what should be the total output during the 11-7 shift?

    (A) 420 cc (ml)

    (B) 860 cc (ml)

    (C) 620 cc (ml)

 *(D) 680 cc (ml)

THE ANSWERS

All the possible choices that could answer the problem presented in the stem are called **answers**. Although the number of answers can vary among tests, the usual number of answers is four. Four answers reduce guessing, while keeping the amount of reading to a reasonable level. Answers are usually identified by numbers (1, 2, 3, and 4), capital letters (A, B, C, and D), or lowercase letters (a, b, c, and d). Of the four answers, only one is the **correct answer**, while the other three are **wrong answers**. Answers can be the completion of the sentence begun in the item, a complete sentence, or an incomplete sentence.

When an answer completes the sentence begun in the stem

When an answer is the completion of the statement begun in the stem, the stem and the answer together should form a grammatically correct sentence that ends with a period.

_____ EXAMPLE 1

Women tend to get urinary infections more often than men because:
- (A) Women cannot use a urinal when voiding.
- (B) The urine flows toward the rectum when voiding.
- (C) Women use bedpans, which tend to grow bacteria.
- *(D) The rectum is closer to the urinary opening.

_____ EXAMPLE 2

The rate of growth and development over the life span can be described as:
- *(A) Uneven.
- (B) Complex.
- (C) Slow.
- (D) Fast.

_____ EXAMPLE 3

During a bed bath the NA can improve a resident's circulation by:
- (A) Using cool water for the bath.
- (B) Putting soap on the washcloth.
- *(C) Using firm strokes toward the heart.
- (D) Keeping the window open during the bath.

When an answer is a complete sentence

When an answer is a complete sentence by itself, it should be a grammatically correct sentence that ends with a period.

_____ **EXAMPLE 1**

What is the first step in a bladder retraining program?
- (A) Find out the resident's usual voiding pattern.
- (B) Offer the resident the bedpan every two hours.
- *(C) Make sure the resident can cooperate.
- (D) Give enough fluids to the resident.

_____ **EXAMPLE 2**

The NA notes that a resident who usually talks a lot is being very quiet. What should the NA say?
- (A) "How come you are so quiet today?"
- (B) "You must be upset about something."
- (C) "What is wrong with you?"
- *(D) "You seem very quiet today."

_____ **EXAMPLE 3**

What should the NA do to prevent residents from getting burned while smoking?
- (A) Allow residents only one cigarette per hour.
- *(B) Supervise residents when they smoke.
- (C) Keep all cigarettes away from residents.
- (D) Light cigarettes for all residents.

When an answer is an incomplete sentence

When an answer is an incomplete sentence, it will be a phrase that is not followed by a period.

_____ **EXAMPLE 1**

What is the most often used method for preventing a resident from falling out of bed?
- (A) Wrist restraints
- *(B) Bedside rails
- (C) Sedative medications
- (D) Frequent checking

_____ **EXAMPLE 2**

Besides a sphygmomanometer, what piece of equipment would an NA need to take a person's blood pressure?
- (A) Thermometer
- (B) Glucometer
- (C) Watch
- *(D) Stethoscope

_____ **EXAMPLE** 3

Which of the following is most effective in preventing the spread of infection in a nursing home?

   (A) Isolation
   (B) Antibiotics
   (C) Sterilization
 *(D) Handwashing

SPECIFIC TEST-TAKING SKILLS

Nothing can improve your score more on a test than adequate preparation. Effective studying provides you with an opportunity to memorize facts, understand new information, and learn how to use information in new situations. In addition to understanding the subject being tested, it is also important to be test-wise. Being test-wise is not learning gimmicks or tricks of the trade, but rather how to analyze a test item to increase the chances of getting the item correct.

Each item should be broken down into its parts and examined. First, look at the stem to find out what is being asked. Then, look at the answers to throw out wrong answers logically until you are left with what you think is the correct answer. Some items are easy because you quickly see the correct answer among the four answers. You recognize it as the correct answer based on the information you know and understand. However, do not be tempted to quickly answer the item without looking at it closely. While an answer may contain information that is true, it may not be the correct answer because it is not related to the question being asked. Use your test-taking skills for every item. If you are unsure of the answer, then test-taking skills become more important when trying to throw out wrong answers.

In an item that has four answers, the chance of getting the item correct is one out of four, or 25%. If you are able to throw out one wrong answer, the chance of getting the item correct is one out of three, or 33%. If you are able to throw out two wrong answers, the chance of getting the item correct is one out of two, or 50%. Each time you throw out a wrong answer, you increase your chance of getting the item correct. The following test-taking skills may help you become test-wise and improve your chances of scoring well on a test.

Skill 1—Identify key words in the stem

Read the stem slowly and carefully. Try to identify what the statement is asking. Be alert for key words, such as except, not, and never, that make a negative statement. Look for key words, such as most, least, or first, that modify what is being asked. Often these words are brought to your attention by being **boldfaced**, CAPITALIZED, underlined, "quoted," or *italicized*. When key words such as most important are used, often all four answers are good answers but only one is the best. If the answers do not make sense when you read them, go back and reread the stem to make sure you did not miss a key word.

_____ **EXAMPLE 1**

The *most* important thing to teach a newly admitted resident is:

    *(A) How to use the call bell.
    (B) When meals will be served.
    (C) Why side rails are used.
    (D) Who is in charge of the unit.

A key term in this stem is *most* important. The stem is asking you to place a value on each answer. Each of these answers has something you would teach a newly admitted resident. You must pick the answer that is most important when compared to the other answers. If you are having trouble picking the answer that is most important, rank the answers starting with those you think are least important when a client is admitted. Your choice for the correct answer (most important) would then be the one you listed last.

_____ **EXAMPLE 2**

Which of the following would be LEAST helpful in safely moving a resident from a bed to a wheelchair?

    (A) Keeping the wheels of the wheelchair locked
    (B) Using two people to help with the transfer
    *(C) Placing the wheelchair six feet away from the bed
    (D) Putting shoes on the feet of the resident

A key term in this stem is LEAST helpful. The stem is asking you to place a value on each answer. You must pick the answer that would prove less helpful when compared to each of the other answers. If you are having trouble picking the answer that is least helpful, rank the answers starting with those you think are most helpful for a safe transfer. Your choice for the correct answer (least helpful) would then be the one you listed last.

_____ **EXAMPLE 3**

If a resident chokes on a piece of food and cannot speak, what should the nurse aide do **first**?

    (A) Call the nurse immediately.
    (B) Begin cardiopulmonary resuscitation (CPR).
    (C) Pound three times on the resident's back.
    *(D) Perform the Heimlich maneuver.

A key term in this stem is **first**. The stem is asking you to set a priority. You must decide what is the most important thing to do in this situation before anything else.

Skill 2—Focus on the person

Your job as an NA is concerned with providing physical and emotional care to people. Test items are trying to find out if you know how to care for people both physically and emotionally. Therefore, when you look at the answers, carefully look at the ones that focus on the resident or are directed at feelings.

_____ **EXAMPLE 1**

A resident had pain yesterday. Whom should the NA talk with to find out if he is in pain today?
   (A) The nurse
  *(B) The resident
   (C) The doctor
   (D) The roommate

This question is asking you how you would get information about how someone feels. Pain is a personal, subjective feeling. The resident is the best person to talk with to find out if he is still having pain. To answer this question, you had to focus on the resident.

_____ **EXAMPLE 2**

The NA helps a resident who has an above-the-knee amputation into a wheelchair. The resident starts to cry and says, ''What good am I with this leg chopped off!'' What should the NA say?
   (A) ''It wasn't chopped off, you had an operation.''
   (B) ''You can still stand on your other leg.''
  *(C) ''It must be hard to adjust to losing a leg.''
   (D) ''You'll feel better when you get a new wheelchair.''

In this question the resident is sharing a feeling with the NA. He is crying and feels worthless. The resident needs to feel accepted and have a chance to talk. All of the wrong answers deny feelings and cut off communication. The correct answer focuses on the resident by talking about how hard it must be for him.

_____ **EXAMPLE 3**

When styling a female resident's hair, what should the NA do first?
  *(A) Ask the resident how she would like it styled.
   (B) Start at the roots using long, even strokes.
   (C) Use alcohol to untangle the matted areas.
   (D) Part the hair down the back and make two pigtails.

How a person combs the hair is a very personal choice and reflects a person's individual identity. Therefore, when you look at the answers, carefully look at the ones that focus on the resident or expect the resident to make a choice. Answers B, C, and D focus on physical actions done by the NA. Answer A is the only answer that focuses on the resident.

Skill 3—Identify specific clues

The stem is usually short and has only the information needed to make it clear and exact. A specific clue is a word (or words) in the stem that provides a hint for choosing the correct answer. The word in the stem that is a specific clue may be the same as (identical) or similar to the word in the correct answer. Look for words that are the same or closely related when looking at the stem and the answers.

_____ **EXAMPLE 1**

Which of the following actions would meet a resident's basic physical needs?
- (A) Talking with the resident
- (B) Putting up side rails
- (C) Admiring a sweater
- *(D) Giving physical hygiene

Physical needs are important words in this stem. When looking at the answers, one of them contains the word **physical**. Carefully look at this answer. More often than not it will be the correct answer.

_____ **EXAMPLE 2**

What is the main reason for range of motion exercises?
- *(A) Keeps joints moving
- (B) Limits muscle tone
- (C) Prevents bedsores
- (D) Helps breathing

Range of motion exercises are important words in this stem. When looking at the answers, one of them contains the word **moving**. The words motion and moving are similar. Be alert and closely look at this answer. It may be a clue that it is the correct answer.

_____ **EXAMPLE 3**

The main reason you rinse a resident's skin during a bath is to:
- (A) Improve circulation.
- *(B) Remove soap.
- (C) Cool the resident.
- (D) Prevent pressure sores.

Rinse is an important word in this stem. When looking at the answers, one of them contains the word **remove**. The words rinse and remove are similar. Be alert and closely look at this answer. It may be a clue that it is the correct answer.

Skill 4—Identify similar/different answers

Sometimes an item will contain two or more answers that are a lot alike. Usually when two answers are similar, they are wrong answers. When you find similar answers, you can throw them both out. The correct answer will then be one of the two answers that are left. By throwing out two wrong answers, you have increased your chance of getting the item right to 50%. When three answers are similar, you can throw all of them out and the remaining answer, which is different, is frequently the correct answer.

_____ **EXAMPLE 1**

What is the **most** important thing the NA should do when moving a person from a bed to a wheelchair?

  *(A) Provide for the safety of the resident.
   (B) Lock the wheels on the bed and the wheelchair.
   (C) Report to the charge nurse after the transfer.
   (D) Get another NA to help with the transfer.

Answers B and D are specific things that could be done to ensure a safe transfer. Both are equally important, and it would be hard to choose one as the correct answer over the other. Now look at the other answers. Answer C would be done after, not during, the transfer and therefore can be thrown out. That leaves answer A as the correct answer. Answer A actually includes answers B and D because both these actions provide for the safety of the resident during the transfer. Answer A is more complete and includes the others.

_____ **EXAMPLE 2**

The NA finds Mrs. Jones in bed with her eyes closed. Which of the following conclusions should be made by the NA?

   (A) She is feeling withdrawn.
  *(B) The NA needs more information.
   (C) Mrs. Jones is unconscious.
   (D) The resident is sleeping.

Answers A, C, and D are similar. They all come to a conclusion about the resident's physical or emotional state. Answer B is different from the others.

_____ **EXAMPLE 3**

A resident is upset and goes into a long discussion about something that happened yesterday. What should the NA do?

  *(A) Listen for causes of the problem.
   (B) Give an opinion about the problem.
   (C) Tell her to tell you what is wrong.
   (D) Interrupt and try to calm her down.

Answers B, C, and D all require the NA to talk. Answer A requires the NA to listen. This is different from the other possible answers. Many times the correct answer is different from the other possible answers.

Skill 5—Identify answers with absolute terms

Carefully read each answer. Look for key words such as **always, never, all, every,** and **none.** These terms are absolute and have no exceptions. They place special limits on a statement that might otherwise be correct. Answers with these words in them are usually not the correct answer and can be thrown out. By eliminating one wrong answer, the chance of your choosing the correct answer is 33% rather than 25%. You have increased your chances of getting the answer correct.

_____ **EXAMPLE 1**

When should a comb or brush be washed?
  (A) Every time it is used
  (B) Once a day
  *(C) Whenever the hair is washed
  (D) Once a month

In answer A the word **every** is an absolute term. This word allows for no exceptions. Every time a comb or brush is used it must be washed, even if it is used six times a day. This would not be practical. By throwing out this wrong answer, you increase your chance of choosing the correct answer because you only have to choose from among three answers rather than four.

_____ **EXAMPLE 2**

Mr. Allen is angry because he can no longer do many things for himself. What should the NA do to make him feel less angry?
  (A) Tell him what he can do.
  (B) Assist him with all of his care.
  (C) Encourage him to accept his dependence.
  *(D) Give him choices about his care.

In answer B the word **all** is an absolute term. It is a strong word that includes everything. An answer that has an absolute term is usually not the correct answer. By throwing out this wrong answer, you increase your chance of getting the item correct.

_____ **EXAMPLE 3**

The main reason the NA positions a resident every two hours is to:
  *(A) Reduce pressure.
  (B) Observe the skin.
  (C) Provide activity.
  (D) Relax all muscles.

In answer D the word **all** is an absolute term. This word allows for no exceptions. When positioning a resident, it may not be possible for the resident to relax all muscles. By throwing out this wrong answer, you increase your chances of getting the item correct because you only have to choose among three answers rather than four.

Skill 6—Identify similar parts in answers

Sometimes answers contain two or more parts that are the same (identical) or similar. If you can identify one part as being incorrect, you can usually throw out two answers. By eliminating two wrong answers, you have reduced the number of answers from which you have to choose the correct answer. You now have a 50% chance of getting the item correct.

_____ **EXAMPLE 1**

Mr. Marshall is holding a lot of fluid in his feet and ankles and is very overweight. What kind of a diet should the NA expect the doctor will order?
  *(A) Low salt, low calorie
  (B) Low salt, low protein
  (C) High salt, low calorie
  (D) High salt, low protein

If you knew that people who hold extra fluid are usually put on a low salt diet, then you could throw out answers C and D. You are left with only two answers from which to choose the correct answer. By throwing out two wrong answers, your chance for getting the item correct is now 50%. Then, if you know that people who are overweight are put on low calorie diets, you can throw out answer B and the correct answer is A.

_____ **EXAMPLE 2**

Which of the following vital signs should be reported to the nurse?
  (A) Pulse rate of 72, oral temperature of 99° F
  (B) Pulse rate of 92, respirations of 18 per minute
  (C) Pulse rate of 92, oral temperature of 98.6° F
  *(D) Pulse rate of 102, respirations of 28 per minute

If you knew that the normal range for an oral temperature is between 97.6° and 99.6° F, then you could throw out answers A and C. You are left with only B and D from which to choose the correct answer. You have increased your chance to choose the correct answer to 50%. To choose between answers B and D you would not have to know the normal range for _both_ the pulse rate and the respiratory rate. If you knew that the normal range for a pulse is between 60 and 100, you could throw out answer B because the pulse rate was within this range. Answer D would then be the correct answer. If you knew that the normal range for respirations was between 14 and 24, you could throw out answer B because the respirations were within this range. Answer D would then be the correct answer. Of course, it is best to know the normal range for all of these vital signs. However, eliminating wrong answers can improve your chance of getting the item correct.

_____ **EXAMPLE 3**

Which of the following signs and symptoms of respiratory distress should the NA immediately report to the nurse?
  (A) Respirations of 14, regular rhythm
  (B) Respirations of 18, shallow breathing
  (C) Respirations of 20, regular rhythm
*(D) Respirations of 34, shallow breathing

If you knew that the normal range for respirations is 14 to 20 breaths per minute, you should immediately pick D as the correct answer. However, if you only knew that respirations should have a regular rhythm, then you could throw out A and C as wrong answers. You would then be left with only B and D from which to choose the correct answer. You have increased your chance to choose the correct answer to 50%. Eliminating two wrong answers has improved your chance of getting the item correct.

Skill 7—Use more than one test-taking skill

You have just learned six specific test-taking skills that should help you increase your chance of correctly answering test items. It is suggested that you study the six test-taking skills so that you fully understand how to apply each of them to the analysis of an item. Depending on how an item is written, you can use more than one test-taking skill when analyzing a test item.

_____ **EXAMPLE 1**

The doctor orders 1,000 cc (ml) of fluid restriction a day. What should the nurse aide do **first**?
  (A) Record the I&O each shift.
  (B) Give fluids just with meals.
  (C) Encourage only clear fluids.
*(D) Put a sign at the bedside stating "restrict fluids."

Answers B and C are similar. They both address giving fluids. A and D are different and should be looked at more closely. This used Skill 4—Identify Similar/Different Answers.

The key word **first** in the stem should clue you to D as the correct answer. To restrict a resident to 1,000 cc (ml) of fluid per day, all team members must be aware that fluids are restricted. The sign must be posted first, then all fluids given can be placed on the I&O record. This used Skill 1—Identify Key Words in the Stem.

_____ **EXAMPLE 2**

Mrs. Penn had a stroke and is not able to move her left arm and leg. When the NA is dressing her, Mrs. Penn starts to cry and says, ''I am useless since I cannot move my arm and leg.'' What should the NA say?

   (A) ''All people who have a stroke feel that way.''
   (B) ''Cheer up. You will be able to move after physical therapy.''
  *(C) ''It must be difficult not being able to move your arm and leg.''
   (D) ''Things will be OK after you start to feel better.''

Answer A includes the word all. By including this word in the sentence, there are no exceptions to the answer. Since all people do not behave or feel the same way, answer A can be thrown out as a wrong answer. This used Skill 5—Identify Answers with Absolute Terms.

Answers B and D both talk about how things will get better in the future. It would be hard to pick one of these over the other as the correct answer. Therefore, these could be thrown out as wrong answers. This used Skill 4—Identify Similar/ Different Answers.

In the stem the use of the words **arm and leg** is a clue for choosing the correct answer. Answer C has the words arm and leg in its statement. Look at this answer closely because it is probably the correct answer. This used Skill 3—Identify Specific Clues.

_____ **EXAMPLE 3**

When doing range of motion (ROM) exercises the NA should NOT move:

  *(A) The resident beyond the point of pain.
   (B) Joints of unconscious residents.
   (C) Paralyzed joints.
   (D) Joints that have arthritis.

A key word in this stem is NOT. This stem is negatively worded. It is trying to find out if you can pick out the one answer that would be the wrong thing to do for a resident. To answer this item, first list the answers that include things that you would do for a resident. The answer that is left should be the correct answer to the item. This used Skill 1—Identify Key Words in the Stem.

Answers B, C, and D all refer to types of joints. These are similar answers. Look at answer A. It talks about when you should stop moving a joint. Answer A is different than the other answers. This used Skill 4—Identify Similar/Different Answers.

_____ **EXAMPLE 4**

A resident has a decubitus. To protect the resident's skin, the NA should encourage her to use a:
*(A) Sheepskin.
 (B) Cane.
 (C) Walker.
 (D) Splint.

Answers B and C are both devices that help a person to walk. It would be hard to choose one over the other as the correct answer. Both of these answers are probably wrong. This used Skill 4—Identify Similar/Different Answers.

Protect the resident's skin are important words in this stem. Answer A contains the word **skin** in **sheepskin.** Closely look at this answer as it may be the correct answer. This used Skill 3—Identify Specific Clues.

_____ **EXAMPLE 5**

An NA will be getting married in two weeks. To involve the resident in the excitement of the wedding, the NA should say:
 (A) "I know you can't go, but I'll bring you pictures."
 (B) "Let me tell you about my wedding plans."
*(C) "Mrs. Shoemaker, tell me about your wedding."
 (D) "I am so excited, I can hardly wait for the big day."

Answers B and D are similar because they focus on the NA. It would be difficult to choose between these two answers and therefore they are probably wrong. This used Skill 4—Identify Similar/Different Answers.

Of the two answers that are left, A and C, only C involves the resident in the excitement of a wedding because she is asked to recall an exciting point in her life. This correct answer focuses on the resident. This used Skill 2—Focus on the Person.

GENERAL TEST-TAKING SKILLS

Skill 1—Get a good night's sleep

Get a good night's sleep the night before the test. Do not be tempted to have an all night cram session the night before the test. This will do more harm then good. Plan an enjoyable activity. For example, take a walk, watch a movie, or spend an evening with the family or friends. A rested mind and body provide the energy needed to take the test.

Skill 2—Be on time

Be on time for the examination. Give yourself extra time to arrive at the testing site. Traffic might be heavy, you may get lost, you could run out of gas, the bus could be late, or the trains may not run on time. Plan ahead so that you arrive at least 30 minutes early. This will give you time to visit the rest room, get a good seat, take out your pen and pencils, and collect your thoughts.

Skill 3—Bring the right tools

Bring the right tools with you to the test. Taking a test is a lot like doing a job. If you have the right tools, the job should be easier. Bring at least two pens, several number 2 pencils, and an eraser. A pen may be needed to fill in the information at the top of the answer sheet. Pencils will be needed to fill in the spaces for the correct answers on the answer sheet. Number 2 pencils have soft lead that is needed for computer scoring of the answer sheets. Sharpen the pencils. Remember, a sharp point makes for a sharp mind! An eraser may be needed to change an answer or erase extra marks that you made on the answer sheet. Bring a watch to help you keep track of your time.

Skill 4—Read all directions carefully

Test instructions are very important and are the ground rules for the test. If the person giving the test (proctor) reads the instructions out loud, read along with the proctor. Do not be tempted to read ahead or rush through them to get to the questions. You must totally understand what the instructions are asking you to do before you move on. If you do not understand the instructions, ask the proctor for help.

Skill 5—Use your time well

Some tests are **speed** tests. These tests have severe time limits, and most test-takers do not finish all the questions on the test. Other tests are **power** tests. These tests usually have more than enough time for most test-takers to answer every question. Power tests try to identify how much knowledge or information the test-taker has. All tests will have a time limit. Some are just more generous than others.

To use your time well, divide the total time you have for the test by the number of questions on the test. This will tell you about how much time you have to answer each question. Always leave a little extra time at the end of the test for review. For example, let's say you have 2 hours (120 minutes) for a test and there are 55 questions. If you divide the 120 minutes by 55 questions, you will have about 2 minutes and 19 seconds to answer each question. Pace yourself so that you do not spend more than 2 minutes on any question. By doing this you will not waste too much time on any one question. If you answer a question in less than 2 minutes, this time can be used for answering other questions that take a little longer than 2 minutes or for adding to the time you have for review. Keep your watch handy. If you figure that you have about 2 minutes a question, then by the time 20 minutes have passed, you should have completed at least 10 questions.

Use all the time you are allowed. If you rush through the test, you may read the questions too quickly, come to hasty conclusions, get careless, or not give the proper attention to details. Haste makes waste! Do not let other people's actions make you nervous or anxious. The test-takers who hand in their papers early may be good test-takers and score high. However, they may have given up or rushed through the test and therefore may score low or not pass the test. Be your own person, use all of the time, and use it well.

Skill 6—Work from easy to hard

Work the easy questions first. When you get to a question that you think is hard and may take longer than 2 minutes to answer, leave it for later. Make a note for yourself so that you know which questions you are skipping. Make a mark in your test booklet if allowed, make a list of the question numbers, or make a light mark on the answer sheet next to the question you skipped. Marking the answer sheet will ensure that you do not make the mistake of marking your answer to the next question in the wrong place. However, if you mark the answer sheet, these marks must be fully erased before handing it to the proctor. Move on to the next question. When you finish the last question, go back and try to answer the questions you saved for the end. This test-taking skill allows you to answer as many questions as possible in the time allowed.

Skill 7—Reduce your anxiety

Reduce your anxiety to an acceptable level. A little bit of anxiety before a test can help you to focus your attention to the task at hand. However, anxiety or panic on the day of the test can cause problems when you are trying to think. Try to reduce your anxiety **before** it gets too high. When you feel yourself getting nervous or anxious, use anxiety reducing skills that work for you. For example, skip the hard questions, close your eyes for a few seconds, take several deep breaths, slowly rotate your head around the shoulders, or keep a positive outlook.

Skill 8—Make educated guesses

Make educated guesses, particularly if there is no penalty for guessing. Some tests give credit if you pick the one correct answer and do not give credit if you pick one of the wrong answers. The instructions for these tests may tell you to answer every question, that only correct answers will be counted, or not to leave any blanks.

In these tests it is to your advantage to answer every question. Use your knowledge to pick the correct answer, reduce the number of possible answers and make an educated guess, or, as a last resort, make a wild guess. You will not be penalized for a wrong answer.

Some tests give credit if you pick the one correct answer and take away credit if you pick one of the wrong answers. The instructions for these tests may tell you not to guess, that points will be deducted for wrong answers, that there is a penalty for guessing, or that guessing will be penalized. In these tests if you can reduce the number of possible answers to two, it is usually to your advantage to make an educated guess. However, wild guessing, such as flipping a coin or closing your eyes and picking an answer, is not to your advantage.

Skill 9—Review your answers

If you have time, review your answers after you complete the test. Sometimes content in one question can provide a clue for answering another question or remind you of information that can help you to make an educated guess to a hard question. Be careful about changing an answer you chose first. Only change an answer if you are certain your first choice was an error.

Skill 10—Check your answer sheet

Check your answer sheet at the end of the test. Most computer scored tests have you mark your answers to all the test questions on a separate answer sheet. The answer spaces are lettered or numbered. When you decide which answer is the correct answer, mark the same letter or number on the answer sheet for that question. Make sure all the marks are heavy and full and are within the lines. Ensure you have answered every question. Erase any extra marks on the answer sheet. Extra pencil marks, poorly erased marks, or marks outside the lines will confuse the computer, and you could get a lower score.

CHAPTER 5

Practice Test for State Nurse Aide Evaluation Programs

In 1987 the federal government of the United States passed the Omnibus Reconciliation Act (OBRA). This act requires the training and competency testing of nurse aides (NAs) in long term care. The requirements for training and testing were designed to assure the public that NAs have at least the minimum skills and knowledge needed to deliver safe care to residents.

According to OBRA, all presently working NAs must pass a state issued testing program by December 31, 1989, and be listed in a state registry to be able to work as an NA in long term care. After December 31, 1989, newly hired NAs will have a specific amount of time from the date of hiring to be trained, tested, and registered in order to work. There is a possibility that the deadline for registration and the deadline for training, testing, and registration of newly hired NAs may be modified. Check with the department of health in your state to find out if there are any changes that might affect your status.

When you meet all the requirements for being an NA, then you can apply for the state testing program. Each state has its own specific requirements. Therefore, you must check with your state department of health for specific details required by your state. Most states are requiring a written test, and some states are also requiring a clinical skills test.

CLINICAL COMPETENCY TEST

If your state tests clinical skills, you can obtain a list of the clinical skills being tested from your state department of health. A clinical skills test usually consists of a sample of procedures from a total list of procedures that you must be able to do correctly. While you do the procedures you are scored by a trained evaluator. In most states if you fail the clinical test, you can take it more than once. However, if you fail the clinical skills test on the last try, you must take or repeat a state approved NA training program before you can reapply for testing.

WRITTEN COMPETENCY TEST

Written test

In most states the written test consists of 50 to 60 multiple choice questions. Each question tests a certain piece of information, knowledge, or principle of NA practice. You must choose the correct answer from four choices. One answer is the correct answer and three answers are wrong. For details on how to take and study for a multiple choice test, see Chapters 2 and 4 of this text.

Most states allow you to take the written test more than once. However, if you fail the written test on the last try, you must take or repeat a state approved NA training program before reapplying for the testing program.

Written test: Oral option

Some states offer the written test in an oral format for NAs who have difficulty reading English. Oral tests are usually given by a tape recording of the written test. You are provided with a copy of the test so that you can read along with the tape recording. In some states if you take the oral option, you must also take a job related reading comprehension test that will test your ability to respond to common oral and written stimuli. If you have difficulty reading English, check with your state department of health to find out if an oral option of the written test is available in your state.

INTRODUCTION TO TEST DRILLS

The following three test drills have been designed to cover similar content and in a similar proportion to that you may find on a state NA written competency test. Find a quiet place to work where you will not be interrupted for the entire time you plan to practice test-taking. Answer forms for each test are provided in the back of this textbook. Use a number 2 pencil when recording your answer on the computer sheet. For each question, darken the space that indicates your choice. Practice staying within the lines when recording your answer. Give yourself about two hours for each test. Pace yourself by spending no more than two minutes on each question. If you spend more than two minutes on a question, then you will have less time to spend on another question. If you are having trouble with a question, skip it and move on to the next question. After you complete all the questions, go back to those with which you had trouble and try to answer them. To learn to pace yourself for the test in your state, call your state department of health and ask how many questions are on the test and how much time you have to complete the test. To find out how much time you have for each question, divide the total amount of time by the total number of questions.

Complete and review your answers one test at a time. This allows you to test your growth from one test to the next. When you have completed a test, check your answers against the correct answers. Read the reason for the correct answer. Then read the reasons why the wrong answers are incorrect. Pay special attention to those answers you got wrong. Try to figure out why you chose the wrong answer. For example, did you not know the information, did you read the stem incorrectly, or did you jump to an answer too quickly without carefully analyzing the choices? The review of the reasons for the correct and wrong answers should help you to increase your body of knowledge and improve your test-taking ability.

TEST DRILL 1

Questions

1. What must the nurse aide (NA) check to find out what to do for a resident?
   (A) The NA assignment sheet
   (B) The nursing care plan
   (C) The doctor's orders
   (D) The nurse's notes

2. What measurement would be helpful in identifying a problem with nutrition?
   (A) Temperature
   (B) Weight
   (C) Pulse
   (D) Respiration

3. Which of the following should the NA NOT do to promote personal energy?
   (A) Eat breakfast every day.
   (B) Exercise several times a week.
   (C) Get a good night's sleep.
   (D) Drink a lot of coffee.

4. How often should mouth care be given to the unconscious resident?
   (A) Every hour
   (B) Every two hours
   (C) Every shift
   (D) Every day

5. Which of the following actions by the NA would support a resident's right to privacy?
   (A) Speaking in a kind way
   (B) Providing information about care
   (C) Draping the resident for perineal care
   (D) Telling your name to the resident

6. The NA observes that Mr. Jones goes into rooms of other residents without permission. This makes the other residents angry. What should the NA do with this information at the resident care conference?
   (A) Share the observation with the team.
   (B) Suggest that he be kept in his room.
   (C) Be quiet and maintain confidentiality.
   (D) Request that he be restrained in a chair.

7. The NA breaks a resident's dentures because of carelessness. What legal term applies to this action?
   (A) Negligence
   (B) Crime
   (C) Ethics
   (D) Warning

8. What sense is most important to a resident who appears to be in a coma?
   (A) Sight
   (B) Hearing
   (C) Touch
   (D) Smell

9. A resident who is usually very active and happy does not want to get out of bed and seems sad. What should the NA do?
   (A) Ignore the behavior.
   (B) Allow her to stay in bed.
   (C) Report this to the nurse.
   (D) Act happy and tell a joke.

10. Under whom does the NA directly work?
    (A) The doctor
    (B) The charge nurse
    (C) The director of nursing
    (D) The nursing supervisor

11. What should the NA do to be sure that the resident understands what has been said?
    (A) Speak clearly when giving directions.
    (B) Ask the resident to repeat what was said.
    (C) Talk slowly when speaking with the resident.
    (D) Use simple words and sentences.

12. Which of the following would NOT stop hair from tangling and matting?
    (A) Braiding in pigtails
    (B) Daily brushing
    (C) Washing with shampoo
    (D) Using conditioners

13. Mr. West's wife died 2 weeks ago. When talking about her he starts to cry. How should the NA respond?
    (A) Leave the room to provide privacy.
    (B) State, "Try not to cry, things will get better."
    (C) Say, "It must be hard to lose someone."
    (D) Take him to the day room to be with others.

14. Mr. Glass has an infected decubitus and is on drainage/secretion precautions. What should the NA wear in addition to a gown?

    (A) Gloves
    (B) Mask
    (C) Boots
    (D) Hat

15. The NA is taking an extinguisher to a fire scene in response to an alarm. What should the NA do?

    (A) Pull the fire alarm.
    (B) Run as fast as possible.
    (C) Remove the safety pin.
    (D) Use the stairs.

16. When a resident has a seizure, what should the NA do *first*?

    (A) Get a tank of oxygen.
    (B) Put a pillow under the resident's head.
    (C) Hold the resident's arms and legs firmly.
    (D) Move furniture away from around the resident.

17. Mrs. Andrews is crying and the only word the NA hears is daughter. What should the NA say?

    (A) "What are you saying about your daughter?"
    (B) "I'm sure that your daughter is OK."
    (C) "What did your daughter do to upset you?"
    (D) "Do you want your daughter to visit?"

18. A resident dies. When should the NA begin postmortem care?

    (A) When the family arrives
    (B) After death is pronounced
    (C) As soon as the resident stops breathing
    (D) When the nursing supervisor is notified

19. What should the NA say to a person with nasal oxygen to reduce anxiety?

    (A) "This is oxygen, it will help you breathe better."
    (B) "Don't get excited, everything will be all right."
    (C) "If you don't smoke, it will not explode."
    (D) "Don't worry, this is the doctor's orders."

20. A resident is wearing a mitt restraint. How often should the NA release the restraint and massage and exercise the hand?

    (A) Every hour
    (B) Every shift
    (C) Every four hours
    (D) Every two hours

21. Which of the following actions by an NA would NOT meet a resident's emotional needs?

    (A) Assisting a resident to eat
    (B) Explaining what is going to be done
    (C) Calling a resident by name
    (D) Encouraging worthwhile activities

22. Several times a day, every day, a resident asks when bingo will be played. Bingo is played at the same time every day. What should the NA do?

    (A) Explain that she will be taken to bingo every day.
    (B) Tell her that it is at the same time every day.
    (C) Make a sign for her room stating the time for bingo.
    (D) Encourage her to do some other activity.

23. A person on isolation needs a blood pressure reading taken daily. To keep the blood pressure machine (sphygmomanometer) from spreading microorganisms, what should the NA do?

    (A) Keep it at the nurses' station.
    (B) Keep it in a plastic bag.
    (C) Keep it in the dirty utility room.
    (D) Keep it in the resident's room.

24. An unconscious resident begins to vomit while lying on his back in bed. What should the NA do first?

    (A) Sit the resident up.
    (B) Turn the resident on the side.
    (C) Keep the resident flat on his back.
    (D) Take the resident to the bathroom.

25. A resident's vital signs are oral temperature 98.6°, pulse 80, respirations 18, and blood pressure 180/120. Which abnormal sign should the NA immediately report to the nurse?

    (A) Temperature
    (B) Pulse
    (C) Respirations
    (D) Blood pressure

26. Which of the following foods should be encouraged for residents with constipation?

    (A) Milk, creamed soup, and butter
    (B) Bread, nuts, potatoes, and rice
    (C) Fruits, vegetables, and whole grain cereals
    (D) Beef, eggs, and chicken

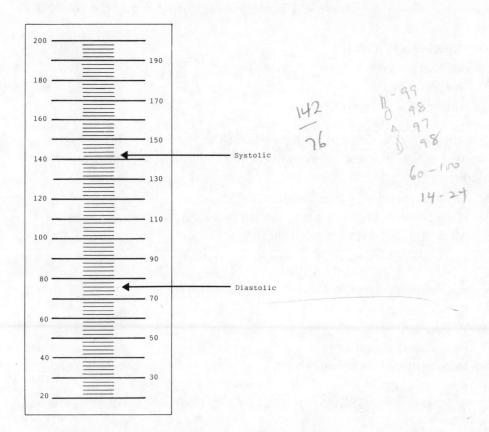

27. The NA took a resident's blood pressure. Using the drawing above, what is the blood pressure?
    (A) 142/76
    (B) 150/80
    (C) 140/70
    (D) 145/75

28. What should the NA do when providing perineal care to a resident with a urinary tube (Foley catheter)?
    (A) Avoid washing the area around the tube.
    (B) Wash down the tube in a circular motion away from the body.
    (C) Wear a gown and sterile gloves throughout the procedure.
    (D) Scrub up and down the tube with soap and water several times.

29. To ensure a successful bladder training program, what is the most important thing the NA should do?
    (A) Offer the resident a full liquid diet.
    (B) Wash the resident's perineal area every shift.
    (C) Tell the nurse when the resident voids.
    (D) Follow the scheduled program exactly.

30. When providing perineal care to a female resident, what should the NA NOT do?
    (A) Pull the curtain closed.
    (B) Wash from back to front.
    (C) Dry skin folds well.
    (D) Rinse the area of soap.

31. A resident must be transferred from a bed to a chair. When being moved to a sitting position, the resident complains that she feels dizzy. What should the NA do?
    (A) Move the resident to the bedside chair quickly.
    (B) Have her stand at the bedside for a few minutes.
    (C) Allow the resident time to sit on the side of the bed.
    (D) Put her head between her knees until she feels better.

32. What is the best way to measure the amount of urine?
    (A) By weight
    (B) With a test tube
    (C) By an accurate guess
    (D) With a marked container

33. A confused resident has trouble finding the day room every day. What should the NA do?
    (A) Take her to the day room every day.
    (B) Make a map for her to follow.
    (C) Assign another resident to take her.
    (D) Plan activities for her in her room.

34. A resident in bed needs a bedpan. What should the NA do to best prevent the resident from falling out of bed?
    (A) Wash the resident's hands before placing the bedpan.
    (B) Raise the side rails on the bed.
    (C) Have the toilet paper ready for use.
    (D) Elevate the head of the bed a little bit.

35. Mr. Taylor has a cold with a high temperature. He sweated (perspired) a lot during the night. What should the NA's plan for hygiene include?
    (A) Providing perineal care only
    (B) Giving a complete bath
    (C) Delaying the bath until later
    (D) Doing a partial bed bath

36. How much fluid should the NAs give a resident during 24 hours to maintain normal fluid balance?

   (A) 500 cc (ml)
   (B) 1,000 cc (ml)
   (C) 2,000 cc (ml)
   (D) 3,000 cc (ml)

37. To check if Mrs. Carney is oriented, what should the NA do?

   (A) Ask her the time, where she is, and her name.
   (B) Ask her who is the president of the United States.
   (C) Check her eyes to see if they follow movement.
   (D) Identify if she can follow simple directions.

38. What is the most important principle to remember when positioning a resident?

   (A) Maintain correct body alignment.
   (B) Make the resident comfortable.
   (C) Elevate the extremities on pillows.
   (D) Keep the head higher than the heart.

39. What can the NA do to prevent burns during mealtime?

   (A) Serve unsteady residents only cold drinks.
   (B) Assist residents with warm coffee if their hands shake.
   (C) Wait until the food is cold before serving it.
   (D) Use plastic instead of metal knives and forks.

NAME:

Activities of Daily Living Flow Sheet																														
MONTH:										YEAR:										DISTRICT:										
1	2	3	4	5	6	7	8	9	10	11	12	13	14	15	16	17	18	19	20	21	22	23	24	25	26	27	28	29	30	31
D																														
E																														
N																														

ELIMINATION: BOWEL   E=Enema   M=Medium BM   C=Colostomy

                            I=Incontinent   S= Small BM   O=No BM

                            L=Large BM

40. A resident has a small bowel movement. When recording this information on the Activity of Daily Living Flow Sheet, which of the following codes would document this resident's bowel movement?

   (A) S
   (B) E
   (C) L
   (D) M

41. A resident shares that he is afraid of the pain he had with his last heart attack. What should the NA do to help the resident deal with this fear?
    (A) Tell him not to worry.
    (B) Listen to the resident's concerns.
    (C) Avoid talking about the pain.
    (D) Administer medication to reduce pain.

42. Mr. Gomez is unconscious and is on a turning schedule. When turning Mr. Gomez the NA sees a small red area on the base of the spine. What should the NA do first?
    (A) Expose the area to the air.
    (B) Apply a warm soak to the area.
    (C) Massage the area with skin lotion.
    (D) Turn the resident every four hours.

43. How can the NA help a resident meet a basic safety and security need?
    (A) Encourage the resident to go to an activity program.
    (B) Place the call bell within easy reach.
    (C) Provide snacks between meals.
    (D) Respect the resident's cultural background.

44. The resident's care includes the use of a water mattress. What must the NA do?
    (A) Ensure that the water does not get too hot.
    (B) Avoid using sharp objects near the bed.
    (C) Make sure that it is plugged into an outlet.
    (D) Pad the mattress to protect it from being soiled.

45. The resident has weak bones because of aging. To help prevent injury to the bones, what should the NA do?
    (A) Provide bath water that is not too hot.
    (B) Give the resident at least 2,500 cc (ml) of fluid daily.
    (C) Apply lotion to the skin every day.
    (D) Turn or move the resident gently.

46. Which of the assigned activities will prevent a resident from getting contractures?
    (A) Encourage the resident to do active range of motion.
    (B) Walk the resident at least once a day in the hall.
    (C) Turn the resident every two hours.
    (D) Have the resident sit in a wheelchair.

47. Mr. Malloney likes to spit his tobacco juice on the floor. What should the NA do *first*?
    (A) Take his chewing tobacco away from him.
    (B) Teach him how to take care of spit safely.
    (C) Keep him in his room until he stops spitting.
    (D) Encourage him to use chewing gum instead of tobacco.

48. The NA makes all of the following assessments. Which should immediately be reported to the nurse because suctioning may be necessary?

   (A) A resident who is short of breath after returning from the bathroom.
   (B) A respiratory rate of 10 breaths per minute by a sleeping resident.
   (C) A resident who is coughing and spitting out a lot of thick mucus.
   (D) A rattling sound in the throat of an unconscious resident.

49. What is the safest way to keep a resident's feet warm?

   (A) Soak them in hot water.
   (B) Put cotton socks on them.
   (C) Lay them on a heating pad.
   (D) Place three blankets over them.

50. The linens of a resident are soiled and wet. When should the NA change the linens?

   (A) On schedule
   (B) Right away
   (C) When requested by the resident
   (D) When directed by the nurse

51. The resident had a stroke and is paralyzed on the left side. When undressing him, what should the NA do?

   (A) Take the clothes off the left side first.
   (B) Get a second person to assist with undressing.
   (C) Remove clothing from the right side before the left.
   (D) Have him stand up to make undressing easier.

52. Mrs. Grey has just been told she has only three months to live. While the NA is giving a bed bath, Mrs. Grey yells that the NA does not know what she is doing. What should the NA do?

   (A) Accept the behavior without getting angry.
   (B) Explain that she is getting good care.
   (C) Avoid the resident for the rest of the day.
   (D) Tell the nurse that the resident wants another NA.

53. Mrs. James, who is paralyzed on the right side because of a stroke, is afraid to be left alone in her room. To help reduce her anxiety, what can the NA do?

   (A) Tell her there are others who also need care.
   (B) Arrange for another resident to stay with her
   (C) Stay with her in her room most of the time.
   (D) Take her to the day room in a wheelchair.

54. Mrs. Glass has a little difficulty swallowing her food. To prevent choking what should the NA do?

    (A) Allow enough time between spoonfuls for chewing.
    (B) Have her drink fluid before swallowing the food.
    (C) Encourage a conversation while she is eating.
    (D) Mash the soft food and take away the hard food.

55. Mrs. Glass has diabetes. Which of the following is a sign of insulin shock that the NA should immediately report to the nurse?

    (A) Thirst
    (B) Dry skin
    (C) Sweating
    (D) Flushed face

TEST DRILL 1

Reasons for answers

The asterisk (*) is in front of the correct answer.

1. *(A) This is written by the charge nurse to direct the NA's actions.
   (B) While the NA can refer to the nursing care plan, it includes more than the NA can legally do for the resident.
   (C) The doctor's orders direct many actions by the nurse who is then responsible for directing the NA by the NA assignment sheet.
   (D) This documents information about the resident and is not used to direct resident care.

2. (A) This measures the body's ability to regulate temperature.
   *(B) Weight loss or gain reflects how well a person is eating.
   (C) Pulse measures heart action.
   (D) This measures the body's ability to breathe air in and out of the lungs; abnormal rates indicate problems with oxygen supply and demand.

3. (A) Food provides calories for energy.
   (B) Exercise increases muscle tone and energy.
   (C) During rest the body repairs itself.
   *(D) Although the caffeine in coffee is a stimulant, it is a drug and if used too much can harm the body.

4. (A) Unnecessary; every two hours is acceptable.
   *(B) Unconscious residents usually mouth breathe, cannot drink fluids, and may receive oxygen. All of these dry the mucous tissue of the mouth; therefore, mouth care should be given every two hours.
   (C) Too long; the mouth can get very dry, causing sores, crusts, and cracking of mucous tissue.
   (D) Same as (C).

5. (A) This supports the resident's right to be treated with consideration and respect, not privacy.
   (B) This supports the resident's right to be given information about treatment and care, not privacy.
   *(C) This supports a resident's right to privacy because very personal care is given in the least embarrassing manner.
   (D) This supports the resident's right to know who is providing care, not privacy.

6. *(A) The NA makes valuable observations about residents that should be shared.
   (B) The resident does not need to be isolated.
   (C) This does not support confidentiality; it also violates other residents' rights for privacy and security.
   (D) This would be holding the resident against his will (false imprisonment), which is illegal.

7. *(A) This is an unplanned wrong that happens as a result of carelessness and a lack of reasonable behavior.
   (B) Breaking a criminal law is a crime; negligence is the breaking of a civil law.
   (C) This is concerned with what is right or wrong behavior.
   (D) This is action that sometimes takes place as a form of punishment handed down by management and is based on facility policy and procedure.

8. (A) An unconscious person's eyes are usually closed or taped closed to protect the eyes from drying.
   *(B) Hearing is believed to be the last sense lost; it is important to talk to all residents.
   (C) Although touch is important, hearing is the most important sense to an unconscious person.
   (D) Smell is the least important sense to the unconscious person.

9. (A) Never ignore changes in behavior.
   (B) This does not address the cause of the behavior.
   *(C) This behavior needs to be assessed more fully by the nurse.
   (D) This would cut off communication and ignore the resident's feelings.

10. (A) The doctor is responsible for medical care, not nursing care.
    *(B) Based on chain of command, the charge nurse is directly responsible for those providing care.
    (C) While the director of nursing service is responsible for the quality of nursing care delivered within the home, this person does not directly supervise the NA on the unit.
    (D) While the supervisor is responsible for the quality of nursing care delivered on several units, this person does not assume direct supervision of the NA on the unit.

11. (A) This helps a person receive information, but it does not help the sender know whether the receiver understood the message.
    *(B) Feedback through words or gestures will let the care giver know whether or not the resident understood the message as intended.
    (C) Same as (A).
    (D) Same as (A).

12. (A) This keeps hair parted in the back and pulled to the side so that it does not tangle.
     (B) This keeps hair in good condition and prevents it from getting tangled beyond correction.
    *(C) This cleans hair but does not untangle hair; hair should be combed and free of tangles before washing.
     (D) This keeps hair feeling silky and slippery, which reduces tangles from forming.

13. (A) This ignores the resident's feelings; it is better to provide an opportunity for residents to talk if desired.
     (B) This denies the resident's feelings and is false reassurance.
    *(C) This focuses on feelings and provides a chance for the resident to talk about his loss.
     (D) This ignores feelings and puts pressure on the resident to socialize with others when he needs time to grieve.

14. *(A) Gown and gloves are needed to protect the uniform and hands which prevents transfer of microorganisms to others.
     (B) Unnecessary; used for respiratory and strict isolation.
     (C) Unnecessary; used in strict isolation.
     (D) Same as (C).

15. (A) Unnecessary; the alarm has already been pulled.
     (B) Unsafe; this can cause panic and accidents.
     (C) This is only done when the extinguisher is actually going to be used.
    *(D) This provides a safe route to the fire because an elevator could break down between floors.

16. (A) Unnecessary; after the seizure the resident should be able to breathe.
     (B) This would bend (flex) the neck, which may block the airway.
     (C) Never restrain movement of arms and legs because this may cause injury.
    *(D) This prevents possible injury by removing objects that the resident could hit during the seizure.

17. *(A) More information is needed to respond correctly to whatever is upsetting the resident.
     (B) This is false reassurance; there is not enough information to come to this conclusion.
     (C) This is a judgment about the daughter that may not be true.
     (D) This is a conclusion based on not enough information.

18. (A) This should not be performed in front of the family.
    *(B) This meets the legal requirements of the law before care can be given to the dead.
     (C) Absence of breathing and heart rate must be checked by a person who is legally responsible.
     (D) This does not meet the legal requirement for pronouncing death.

19. *(A) By hearing what is being done and why it helps to reduce anxiety, the resident gains an understanding of the purpose of the procedure and knowledge reduces fear.
    (B) This is false reassurance and does not convey interest in the resident's feelings.
    (C) This does not explain the purpose of the oxygen; oxygen does not explode, it supports a fire.
    (D) This is false reassurance; it does not explain the purpose of oxygen.

20. (A) Usually every two hours is often enough.
    (B) This is too long a time between release of restraints; most health department codes require that restraints be released every two hours.
    (C) Same as (B).
    *(D) This is often enough for exercise to prevent contractures.

21. *(A) Food, water, sleep, and oxygen meet basic physical needs, not emotional needs.
    (B) This meets a need for safety and security, which are necessary for emotional comfort.
    (C) This meets a need for dignity and self-esteem, which are necessary for emotional comfort.
    (D) Same as (C).

22. (A) This does not answer the question and promotes dependence.
    (B) This does not answer the resident's question about what time bingo is played.
    *(C) This encourages the resident to be independent.
    (D) Bingo is not the problem; memory loss is the problem.

23. (A) Unsafe; this would cause contamination of the nurses' station.
    (B) Unsafe; it would still carry microorganisms to the next resident using the equipment.
    (C) Unsafe; the microorganisms should be kept in the resident's room.
    *(D) This is the most practical because it can be disinfected after the infection is over.

24. (A) Sitting does not prevent vomitus from entering the breathing passages; this action may take too much time or may not be permitted for this resident.
    *(B) This allows vomitus to drain out of the mouth and prevents breathing vomitus into the lungs (aspiration).
    (C) Unsafe; this position makes it very easy for vomitus to enter the breathing passages.
    (D) Unsafe; an unconscious resident cannot be moved to a bathroom.

25. (A) The temperature falls within the normal range of 97.6° to 99.6° F for an oral temperature.
    (B) The pulse falls within the normal range of 70 to 80 beats per minute.
    (C) The respirations fall within the normal range of 14 to 20 per minute.
    *(D) The blood pressure is abnormal; a systolic pressure (the upper number) between 100 and 150 mm Hg is considered normal, and diastolic pressure (the lower number) between 60 and 90 mm Hg is considered normal.

26. (A) Cooked milk is constipating and creamed soup contains milk.
    (B) Nuts are constipating and should be avoided.
    *(C) These foods add bulk, which promotes bowel movements.
    (D) Eggs, especially hard-boiled eggs, are constipating.

27. *(A) Each line has a value of 2 on the blood pressure scale; one line above 140 would be 142; three lines above 70 would be 76.
    (B) Not an accurate reading; both the systolic and the diastolic are too high.
    (C) Not an accurate reading; both the systolic and the diastolic are too low.
    (D) Not an accurate reading; the systolic is too high and the diastolic is too low.

28. (A) The area should be washed with soap and water.
    *(B) This action goes from a clean area (urinary meatus) to a dirty area (down the tubing), which moves soiled material away from the urinary meatus, preventing possible infection.
    (C) A gown is not necessary; this is not a sterile procedure, but clean gloves should be worn to protect the care giver.
    (D) This action moves soiled material toward the urinary meatus and can lead to possible infection.

29. (A) Any type of liquid is helpful to a bladder training program.
    (B) Although important, it will not increase a resident's ability to control voiding.
    (C) Unnecessary; only abnormal patterns should be reported to the nurse; documentation is done on the appropriate form by the NA.
    *(D) The schedule is based on an assessment of the resident's normal pattern; fluid intake is scheduled to increase urinary output when the resident normally voids.

30. (A) Screening provides for privacy and emotional comfort.
    *(B) Incorrect; always wash from front (pubis—clean) to back (rectum—dirty) which moves soiled material away from the urinary meatus and vagina, reducing possible infection.
    (C) This is important because wet, dark, warm areas promote the growth of microorganisms.
    (D) Soap is drying and irritating; therefore, the skin should be well rinsed.

31. (A) Unsafe; the resident is dizzy and could fall.
     (B) Same as (A).
    *(C) When a person moves from lying down to sitting up, blood drains from
         the brain causing dizziness; time is needed for the body to adjust to the
         change in position.
     (D) Same as (A).

32. (A) Weight is not the most accurate way to measure fluid volume.
     (B) A test tube is too small to measure urinary output.
     (C) A guess is never an accurate way to measure fluid volume.
    *(D) A special container with marks indicating cubic centimeters (cc), or
         milliliters (ml), is the most accurate way to measure fluid.

33. *(A) This provides for emotional and physical safety.
     (B) A confused resident could not follow a map.
     (C) Residents should not be responsible for the care of other residents.
     (D) This would isolate the resident.

34. (A) This action does not provide for physical safety.
    *(B) This provides a barrier, to protect the person from falling out of bed, and
         can be held by the resident for balance and comfort.
     (C) This does not provide a barrier to prevent a person from falling out of bed.
     (D) This could cause a person to fall out of bed, especially without a side rail up.

35. (A) This only includes the groin and genital area; the whole body needs to
         be washed.
    *(B) This is necessary because the resident was sweating (perspiring) heavily
         and the skin needs to be cleaned and dried.
     (C) The bath should be done immediately; sweat (perspiration) should not
         stay on the body for long periods of time.
     (D) This only includes the face, hands, and genital area; the whole body needs
         to be washed.

36. (A) This is not enough fluid for survival.
     (B) Same as (A).
    *(C) 2,000 to 2,500 cc (ml) of fluid are needed daily for the body to work
         properly.
     (D) This is more than what is needed daily for normal fluid balance.

37. *(A) Questions concerning time, place, and person are classic for checking
         orientation.
     (B) This is not a good way to check for orientation because the person may
         not be interested in politics or may be oriented but have a problem with
         short term memory.
     (C) A person can do this and still be very disoriented and confused.
     (D) Same as (C).

38. *(A) Correct alignment maintains physical functioning, limits stress on muscles and joints, and prevents contractures.
    (B) While comfort is important, the first and most important goal must be normal alignment.
    (C) Placing pillows under the knees causes them to bend, which can result in contractures if left in this position for long periods of time.
    (D) Unnecessary; the head can be level with the heart.

39. (A) All residents have the right to warm food and drinks; they just need to be assisted.
    *(B) Residents who have mental or physical limitations must be assisted with warm liquids or food to prevent burns.
    (C) Food should be warm, not cold.
    (D) Plastic utensils should only be used in isolation; spilled hot liquids carry a higher risk for causing burns.

40. *(A) S stands for small bowel movement.
    (B) E stands for enema, not small bowel movement.
    (C) L stands for large bowel movement, not small bowel movement.
    (D) M stands for medium bowel movement, not small bowel movement.

41. (A) This denies his feelings.
    *(B) This shows concern and allows him to express his feelings, which may make him feel better.
    (C) This denies feelings and does not give him a chance to discuss his concerns.
    (D) NAs are not licensed to administer medications; the resident is not in pain at this time and does not need pain medication.

42. (A) This requires a doctor's order for treatment.
    (B) This needs a doctor's order and is usually done by the nurse.
    *(C) This helps to increase blood and oxygen to the area.
    (D) The resident should be turned every two hours; the area should be massaged right away.

43. (A) This supports a resident's need for self-esteem.
    *(B) A person usually feels more secure knowing that the use of a call bell will alert someone that they need help.
    (C) This supports a resident's nutritional need, which is a basic physical need.
    (D) This supports a resident's self-esteem needs.

44. (A) Water mattresses are not heated; water beds are heated.
    *(B) Pins or other sharp objects can cause holes in the mattress; when water and air come out of the mattress, it no longer works to limit pressure.
    (C) Water mattresses are not heated and therefore do not need to be attached to a power source.
    (D) This defeats the purpose of the mattress; only one sheet should be between the resident and the mattress.

45. (A) Not related to bone problems; this provides for safety because of decreased ability to feel temperature.
    (B) Not related to bone problems; this may help prevent urinary infections.
    (C) Not related to bone problems; this keeps fluid in the skin, which prevents drying.
    *(D) Calcium leaves the bones as people age (osteoporosis); this weakens the bones and fractures can occur unless people are moved carefully.

46. *(A) Bending (flexing) and opening (extending) joints lengthens muscles, thus preventing contractures.
    (B) Walking does not put all joints through range of motion; this also assumes that the resident can walk.
    (C) This prevents pressure, not contractures.
    (D) Prolonged sitting can cause hip and knee contractures.

47. (A) This would deny the resident's rights; he should be allowed to chew tobacco if infection control guidelines are followed.
    *(B) Tobacco juice and saliva should be put in a waterproof bag; the resident should be allowed to chew tobacco if infection control guidelines are followed.
    (C) This would not stop the spitting; teaching is the first action.
    (D) While this might be done, it does not address the issue of spitting on the floor.

48. (A) Shortness of breath after activity is a sign of lack of oxygen to body tissues, not extra mucus in air passages.
    (B) This is normal; the rate is lower because the need for oxygen is less when activity is decreased.
    (C) A person does not need to be suctioned when able to cough up and spit out mucus (expectorate).
    *(D) The rattling sound in the throat is mucus; an unconscious person cannot cough to rid the air passages of mucus.

49. (A) Feet can be soaked in warm (105 F) water; this is done to clean them, not warm them.
    *(B) The socks trap body heat, which helps to keep the feet warm.
    (C) Unsafe; this could cause tissue injury; heat treatments require a doctor's order.
    (D) This would put too much pressure on top of the feet, causing pointing of the toes and foot-drop.

50. (A) Unsafe; the resident may have to lie in soiled linen for a long period of time.

   *(B) Wet or soiled linens should be changed immediately because they are uncomfortable, allow the growth of microorganisms, cause skin breakdown, and promote infection.

   (C) Some residents may not have the mental ability to know when the bed is wet or soiled.

   (D) This is within the job description of the NA; the NA does not have to wait to be told by a nurse to change the bed.

51. (A) This puts too much stress on the affected side; it is less stressful to take clothing off the unaffected side first.

   (B) Not necessary; one person would be enough to assist with undressing.

  *(C) This puts less stress on the affected side; the unaffected side can move to assist with undressing.

   (D) Unsafe; the resident is paralyzed on the left side and therefore would have to stand on one leg.

52. *(A) The resident's behavior is a reaction to the news of her future death; anger is a defense or reaction to loss.

   (B) Although this may be true, the resident's anger has nothing to do with the NA's care.

   (C) This would isolate the resident at a time when she may need to talk with someone.

   (D) This is an attempt by the NA to avoid the resident.

53. (A) This denies the resident's feelings and may make her feel guilty.

   (B) Residents should not be responsible for other residents.

   (C) Impractical; this would prevent others from getting the care they need from the NA.

  *(D) Keeping her in the middle of activity with others may help her feel less alone and afraid.

54. *(A) Time is needed for chewing to break food down into small pieces mixed with saliva for safe swallowing.

   (B) This could flush food down the airway to the lungs rather than down the esophagus to the stomach.

   (C) She should not talk with food in her mouth because it could cause food to get caught in the air passages.

   (D) Food sometimes needs to be mashed, but the rough texture of food and chewing can be good for the mouth; removal of food would result in the resident not getting adequate nutrition.

55. (A) This is a sign of diabetic coma, not insulin shock.

   (B) Same as (A).

  *(C) This is a classic sign of shock, especially insulin shock.

   (D) Same as (A).

TEST DRILL 1

Answer key

1. A
2. B
3. D
4. B
5. C
6. A
7. A
8. B
9. C
10. B
11. B
12. C
13. C
14. A
15. D
16. D
17. A
18. B
19. A
20. D
21. A
22. C
23. D
24. B
25. D
26. C
27. A
28. B
29. D
30. B
31. C
32. D
33. A
34. B
35. B
36. C
37. A
38. A
39. B
40. A
41. B
42. C
43. B
44. B
45. D
46. A
47. B
48. D
49. B
50. B
51. C
52. A
53. D
54. A
55. C

TEST DRILL 2

Questions

1. A resident is crying. What should the NA say?
   - (A) "Things will be better tomorrow."
   - (B) "Don't cry, it will make you sad."
   - (C) "Would you like to talk about it?"
   - (D) "Cheer up, it is a beautiful day."

2. What is the most important action by the NA when washing the perineal area of a male resident?
   - (A) Washing from the rectum toward the pubis
   - (B) Returning the foreskin over the head of the penis
   - (C) Washing down the shaft of the penis toward the tip
   - (D) Spreading the legs and washing between the labia

3. A resident has severe constipation and may have an impacted stool. The NA should observe for:
   - (A) Small amounts of liquid stool.
   - (B) Bad odor to the breath.
   - (C) Nausea and vomiting.
   - (D) Soft, formed stools.

4. To help a resident meet self-esteem needs, what should the NA do?
   - (A) Dress the resident in neat, clean clothes.
   - (B) Apply a restraint while in a wheelchair.
   - (C) Provide food that the resident likes.
   - (D) Administer oxygen when ordered by the doctor.

5. A resident dies and the family is coming to view the body. What part of the postmortem care should the NA NOT do before the family arrives?
   - (A) Cover the body to the shoulders with a sheet.
   - (B) Gather personal belongings for the family.
   - (C) Secure a chin strap under the chin.
   - (D) Bathe soiled body areas with water.

6. What should the NA do with a resident's blanket that is still clean?
   - (A) Fold it and place it on the back of a chair.
   - (B) Gather it and put it on the overbed table.
   - (C) Store it on the floor of the closet.
   - (D) Replace it with a new blanket from the linen room.

7. Which of the following should the NA do to avoid unpleasant body odor?

  (A) Keep nails short.
  (B) Bathe every day.
  (C) Brush hair daily.
  (D) Clean shoes often.

8. Which of the following pieces of linen is least likely to be reused for the same resident?

  (A) Mattress pad
  (B) Wool blanket
  (C) Bedspread
  (D) Draw sheet

9. The resident tells the NA that her new sweater is missing. What should the NA do?

  (A) Explain that the staff did not take it.
  (B) Tell her that it is in the laundry.
  (C) Report the fact that it is missing.
  (D) Tell her that she does not need it.

10. A resident is having nausea. What should the NA do?

  (A) Provide a liquid diet at mealtime.
  (B) Serve meals and snacks as usual.
  (C) Avoid foods that are high in calories.
  (D) Ask the nurse for directions.

11. An NA gives a resident a bed bath. Which of the following observations should the NA report to the nurse?

  (A) Dry skin
  (B) Gray pubic hair
  (C) Freckles on the back
  (D) Purple-colored heels

12. All of the following are observed by the NA when giving mouth care to an unconscious resident. Which is the *most* serious problem that requires action right away?

  (A) Saliva drooling out of the mouth
  (B) Crusts that have formed on the tongue
  (C) A gurgling sound when breathing
  (D) Sores on the sides of the gums

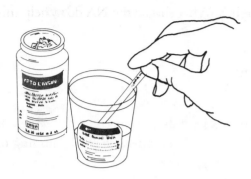

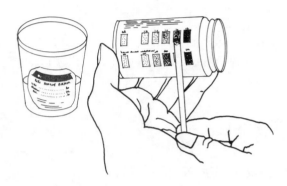

13. What will the NA measure by using the equipment shown above?

    (A) Sugar and acetone of urine
    (B) Microorganisms in the urine
    (C) Amount and color of urine
    (D) Stones in the urine

14. While the NA is giving an enema, the resident says that he has some cramping. What should the NA do?

    (A) Turn the resident on the other side.
    (B) Quickly run in the rest of the fluid.
    (C) Stop the fluid for a few minutes.
    (D) Have the resident bend (flex) the knees.

15. Mrs. Cohen wakes up in the middle of the night and complains of being short of breath. What should the NA do *first*?

    (A) Raise the head of her bed.
    (B) Give her some oxygen.
    (C) Turn her on the side.
    (D) Move her to a chair.

16. Mrs. Allen has dry skin because of aging. What should the NA do to help this problem?
    (A) Tell her to take a bath every day.
    (B) Dress her in a short sleeve blouse.
    (C) Encourage her to sit in the sun.
    (D) Apply lotion after a bath.

17. The NA gets the work assignment from the charge nurse at the beginning of the shift. What should the NA remember to do?
    (A) Do everything that is assigned by the nurse.
    (B) Be friends with the health team workers.
    (C) Know the limits of the NA job description.
    (D) Work without supervision by the nurse.

18. The NA is helping a resident to ambulate. The resident begins to sink to the floor. What should the NA do?
    (A) Lower him to the floor.
    (B) Yell for extra help.
    (C) Hold him up.
    (D) Get him a chair.

19. A newly admitted resident with a urinary catheter needs perineal care. What is the best thing an NA can say?
    (A) "I'm going to wash your Foley catheter."
    (B) "I'm going to wash your urinary meatus."
    (C) "I'm going to wash your private area."
    (D) "I'm going to let you wash your own genitals."

20. When Mr. Deegan lies on his back, his right leg and hip rotate outward from the body (external rotation). Which of the following pieces of equipment should the NA use to prevent external rotation?
    (A) Footboard
    (B) Trochanter roll
    (C) Bed cradle
    (D) Eggcrate mattress

21. An alert resident is recovering from a stroke. What is the best way to position his weak hand?
    (A) In a hard hand splint made by the NA
    (B) Around a hand roll with the fingers slightly flexed
    (C) In a sling supporting the elbow and wrist
    (D) By his side in a mitt restraint

22. The resident asks for advice on a personal matter. What should the NA do?
    (A) Give an opinion about what to do.
    (B) Tell the resident to ask her friends.
    (C) Make believe the question was not heard.
    (D) Ask what the resident thinks.

23. A resident has a colostomy. What should his care include?
    (A) Making sure he gets his special diet
    (B) Limiting his activity to a wheelchair
    (C) Offering him extra fluids throughout the day
    (D) Planning more time for hygiene care

24. To best understand what a resident is saying, what should the NA do?
    (A) Use touch.
    (B) Listen carefully.
    (C) Show interest.
    (D) Be silent.

25. When a resident has just had a cigarette, how long should the NA wait to take an oral temperature?
    (A) 2 minutes
    (B) 5 minutes
    (C) 15 minutes
    (D) 60 minutes

26. To provide for emotional comfort when giving perineal care, what should the NA do?
    (A) Pull the curtain around the bed.
    (B) Position the resident on the back.
    (C) Wash the perineal area well.
    (D) Turn the resident to wash the rectal area.

27. Residents with chronic pain have emotional (psychological) reactions. Which of the following is a psychological reaction for which the NA should observe?
    (A) Increased blood pressure
    (B) Depression
    (C) Increased pulse
    (D) Nausea

28. Which of the following should NOT be used to clean the mouth of an unconscious resident?
    (A) A finger wrapped in a washcloth
    (B) A tongue blade wrapped with gauze
    (C) A lemon and glycerine swab
    (D) A disposable sponge on a stick

29. The resident tells the NA that she wants her bath in the evening. What should the NA do with this information?

    (A) Tell the other NAs about what the resident wants.
    (B) Write it on the NA assignment sheet.
    (C) Tell the nurse so it can be put on the care plan.
    (D) Get an order from the doctor for an evening bath.

30. Which of the following is NOT part of the procedure for making an occupied bed?

    (A) Explaining the procedure to the resident
    (B) Checking bed linen for personal items
    (C) Closing the curtain when making the bed
    (D) Returning unused linen to the linen room

31. A resident with one-sided weakness needs help transferring to a chair. To do this safely, what should the NA do?

    (A) Hold the resident by the arms.
    (B) Use a gait belt for the transfer.
    (C) Have the resident stay in bed.
    (D) Use a walker to help with the transfer.

32. The fire code bell rings in the facility. What is the first thing the NA should do?

    (A) Check the code chart to locate the fire.
    (B) Take an extinguisher to the fire scene.
    (C) Move residents to the day room.
    (D) Pull the fire alarm immediately.

33. Mr. Katz has several periods of angry behavior a week and bothers other residents. He starts to shout at another resident. What should the NA say?

    (A) "Go to your room now."
    (B) "Stop what you are doing."
    (C) "Please sit down and behave."
    (D) "Let's go for a walk."

34. During a bed bath, how can the NA best keep the resident from getting a chill?

    (A) Give a hot drink before the bath.
    (B) Expose only the area being washed.
    (C) Use firm strokes toward the heart.
    (D) Put on a heat lamp during the bath.

35. A resident has tangled and matted hair. What should the NA do?

    (A) Cut out the knots with a scissor.
    (B) Part the hair and braid it.
    (C) Comb a small section at a time.
    (D) Use a small-toothed comb.

36. To reduce burns to the resident's mouth because of very hot food, what should the NA do?

    (A) Put a finger on the food to test its temperature.
    (B) Wait a short time for the hot food to cool.
    (C) Mix the hot food with cold food to cool it down.
    (D) Blow on the hot food to cool it faster.

37. A mentally retarded adult resident is in a self-grooming training program. To increase learning, what would be the *best* action by the NA?

    (A) Praise the resident when goals are met.
    (B) Withhold desserts when goals are not met.
    (C) Ignore the resident when goals are not met.
    (D) Use cigarettes for a reward when goals are met.

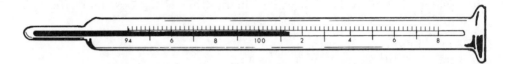

38. What temperature should the NA record from the illustration above?

    (A) 100.6° F
    (B) 101.4° F
    (C) 102.2° F
    (D) 102.6° F

39. Which of the following is the NA legally able to do?

    (A) Transfer and move residents.
    (B) Give medication by mouth.
    (C) Perform a simple sterile dressing.
    (D) Shut off a tube feeding.

40. A resident is receiving oxygen. During the bath the resident's respirations are 34 and she is short of breath. What should the NA do?

    (A) Plan for rest periods during the bath.
    (B) Give a complete bath as fast as possible.
    (C) Give a partial bath and skip the rest of the bath.
    (D) Immediately tell the charge nurse.

41. What should the NA do to prevent injury when applying a wrist restraint?

    (A) Make the wrist strap tight.
    (B) Tie the strap to the bedrail.
    (C) Pad the wrist with something soft.
    (D) Release the restraint every four hours.

42. A resident's daughter has just died. The resident says, "I can't believe my daughter is dead." How should the NA respond?

   (A) Touch her shoulder and say, "I am so sorry."

   (B) Say, "Don't worry, it will be all right."

   (C) Leave the room quickly and quietly.

   (D) State, "I'm sure they tried to help her."

43. Mrs. Jones can use the bathroom safely by herself. To prevent infection, what should the NA teach her to do?

   (A) Take antibiotics four times a day.

   (B) Use her walker to go to the bathroom.

   (C) Wash her hands after toileting.

   (D) Wipe herself from back to front.

44. The resident has dirty feet. To clean them, what is the *best* thing the NA should do?

   (A) Apply lotion to soften the dirt.

   (B) Encourage the resident to take a shower.

   (C) Wipe the feet with cool water and dry well.

   (D) Soak each foot in a basin with soap and water.

45. The NA assignment sheet tells the NA to give a resident passive range of motion (ROM) exercises. What should the NA do?

   (A) Watch the resident do ROM.

   (B) Place the joints in normal body position.

   (C) Move the resident's joints through ROM.

   (D) Take the resident to physical therapy for ROM.

46. A resident has not been eating all of her meals. To measure if her nutritional needs are being met, what should the NA do?

   (A) Take her blood pressure.

   (B) Measure her weight.

   (C) Assess her respirations.

   (D) Count her pulse.

47. When directing a very confused resident with Alzheimer's disease to eat, what should the NA say?

   (A) "Please eat your meat."

   (B) "What would you like to eat?"

   (C) "It's important that you eat."

   (D) "If you don't eat, you can't have dessert."

48. A resident is in a Geri-chair in the day room. She begins to have a seizure. What should the NA do first?

    (A) Apply a jacket and wrist restraint.
    (B) Roll the Geri-chair out of the day room.
    (C) Move the resident to the floor.
    (D) Return the resident to her bed.

49. The resident does not recognize the NA from one day to the next and asks, "Who are you?" What should the NA say?

    (A) "My name is Mary Jones and I will take care of you."
    (B) "I'm the NA. Don't worry, everyone forgets sometime."
    (C) "You know who I am. I took care of you yesterday."
    (D) Say nothing, because it would only upset the resident more.

50. The NA is placing a resident in a mechanical lift tub (Century tub). When the chair is three feet off the ground the resident begins to panic and scream. What should the NA do?

    (A) Continue slowly while saying, "Relax, calm down."
    (B) Lower the chair to the floor right away.
    (C) Stop the chair until the resident calms down.
    (D) Raise the chair quickly and say, "It's almost over."

51. A resident is walking to the day room. She complains of sudden chest pain. What should the NA do *first*?

    (A) Take the resident's vital signs.
    (B) Walk the resident back to her room.
    (C) Get a chair so the resident can rest.
    (D) Monitor the resident's blood pressure.

52. A resident does not respond when spoken to and appears to be sleeping. What should the NA do *first*?

    (A) Tell the charge nurse immediately.
    (B) Say to the resident, "Squeeze my hand."
    (C) Touch the resident gently and call by name.
    (D) Call the resident's name and say, "Wake up."

53. Which of the following actions would be common to all bladder training programs?

    (A) Toileting at 10 AM, 2 PM, 6 PM, and 10 PM
    (B) Toileting as soon as the resident wakes up
    (C) Toileting every four hours and through the night
    (D) Toileting every two hours around the clock

54. Which of the following actions by a resident should be reported to the nurse because the resident might need a restraint?

(A) Wandering around the unit
(B) Falling asleep when in bed
(C) Walking into other resident's rooms
(D) Climbing over the side rail

55. The NA must take a resident's blood pressure and pumps up the cuff. When opening the pressure valve, the gauge drops quickly and the blood pressure reading is not heard. What should the NA do?

(A) Wait two minutes before pumping up the cuff again.
(B) Tell the charge nurse that the machine is broken.
(C) Feel for the pulse on the inside of the elbow.
(D) Clean the earpiece of the stethoscope with alcohol.

TEST DRILL 2

Reasons for Answers

The asterisk (*) is in front of the correct answer.

1. (A) This is false reassurance.
   (B) This denies the resident's feelings; the resident is already sad.
   *(C) This recognizes feelings and gives a chance to share concerns.
   (D) This does not accept the resident's feelings or the need to cry.

2. (A) Incorrect; always wash from clean to dirty; the rectal area is done last.
   *(B) Unless covered by the foreskin, the head of the penis can swell and become painful.
   (C) Washing the penis starts at the tip in a circular motion and continues down the shaft toward the body; this supports the principle of washing from clean to dirty areas.
   (D) A male resident does not have labia; women have labia.

3. *(A) A fecal impaction is an obstruction; stool being pushed around the obstruction becomes very loose.
   (B) This is unrelated to fecal impaction.
   (C) People who need to have a bowel movement may feel bloated or nauseated, but they usually do not vomit.
   (D) This is a normal stool, not a stool of someone with constipation.

4. *(A) How one looks affects a person's self-esteem.
   (B) This meets the resident's need for security and safety.
   (C) This helps to meet a resident's basic physiological need for nutrition and provides choices.
   (D) This helps to meet a resident's basic physical need for oxygen.

5. (A) This provides for dignity.
   (B) This is considered part of postmortem care; the family has a right to receive their family member's belongings.
   *(C) This would be upsetting for the family; the body should be placed in a natural position for viewing.
   (D) This removes odors and cleans the body for viewing.

6. *(A) Gentle folding is the best way to control the spread of microorganisms; the back of a chair is the least contaminated place to store this blanket when not in use.
   (B) A gathered, instead of folded, blanket may fall off a table; an overbed table is considered contaminated.
   (C) This would soil and contaminate the blanket.
   (D) If a blanket is clean, it is not necessary to wash it every time the linen is changed.

7. (A) This will reduce the collection of microorganisms under the nails, not limit body odor.
   *(B) This removes dirt, microorganisms, and sweat (perspiration) from the skin and is the most effective way to prevent body odor.
   (C) Although this helps to keep hair healthy, it will not reduce body odor.
   (D) Cleaning the outside of shoes will not reduce odor; the inside of shoes are rarely cleaned; powder may be applied to the feet to limit foot odor.

8. (A) Unless soiled, this is not changed every time the linen is changed.
   (B) Same as (A).
   (C) Same as (A).
   *(D) This comes in contact with the buttocks; it is the most easily soiled and usually has to be replaced more often than other linens.

9. (A) Although this may be true, it does not solve the problem of the missing sweater.
   (B) This may not be true and is false reassurance.
   *(C) A search and/or investigation cannot begin until the sweater is reported missing.
   (D) This minimizes her feelings and does not recognize her loss.

10. (A) This should not be done without direction from the nurse.
    (B) Same as (A).
    (C) Same as (A).
    *(D) The nausea should be reported to the nurse and directions obtained from the nurse.

11. (A) This is expected with aging.
    (B) Same as (A).
    (C) This is a type of normal skin.
    *(D) This may be the beginning of skin breakdown due to pressure.

12. (A) A correct response to mouth care; the saliva is coming out of the mouth away from the breathing passages.
    (B) Although mouth care should be done more often, this is not an emergency.
    *(C) This is due to fluid in the breathing airway; an unconscious resident will need to be suctioned to remove the fluid that is blocking the air passages.
    (D) Same as (B).

13. *(A) This is a Keto-diastix, which measures sugar and acetone in urine; the results are used to adjust the medication or diet of people with diabetes.
    (B) Keto-diastix does not test for microorganisms; this would need a urine specimen sent to the laboratory for culture.
    (C) A marked container measures urine volume, and observation would note the color of urine.
    (D) Strainers are used to collect stones in the urine.

14. (A) The use of muscles to turn over would probably cause the person to lose control of the fluid already in the intestines.
    (B) This action would make the cramping worse.
    *(C) This stops the pressure of more fluid in the intestine, which decreases cramping.
    (D) This would put pressure on the lower abdomen and probably cause the person to lose control of the fluid already in the intestine.

15. *(A) Sitting up makes breathing easier because it allows the diaphragm to move down with gravity and expand the chest.
    (B) This is the role of the nurse, not the NA.
    (C) It is harder for the lungs to expand when a person is lying flat than when sitting up.
    (D) This would take too much energy when the resident is already short of breath.

16. (A) Bathing would make the problem worse; soap and water are irritating and drying.
    (B) This would not help dry skin.
    (C) This could cause a sunburn and further dry the skin.
    *(D) Lotion helps to keep fluid in the skin, which limits drying.

17. (A) The NA can respectfully refuse to do tasks assigned that are outside the legal limits of the NA job description.
    (B) Health team members should have a courteous and professional relationship; they do not have to be friends.
    *(C) The NA should know exactly what is included on the NA job description and do only those that have been learned and assigned.
    (D) While the NA must be self-directed, the NA works under the direct supervision of the nurse.

18. *(A) Guiding the resident to the floor will help break the fall and limit injury.
    (B) Yelling will only scare the resident and other people in the area; by the time someone comes, the resident will already be on the floor.
    (C) This could hurt the NA or result in both the NA and resident falling.
    (D) Never leave a resident who is falling; always stay and guide the resident to the floor.

19. (A) Most people do not understand technical terms.
    (B) Same as (A).
  *(C) Most people understand that private areas mean the genitals between the legs; later the NA can relate private areas to perineal area.
    (D) Residents should not do perineal care on themselves if they have a urinary tube (Foley).

20. (A) This prevents foot-drop, not external rotation.
  *(B) This holds the hip and leg in normal body alignment and prevents external rotation of the leg and hip.
    (C) This holds the blankets and sheets off the lower legs and feet to prevent foot-drop and discomfort, not external rotation.
    (D) This is used to prevent a decubitus, not external rotation.

21. (A) Splints are usually ordered by the doctor and professionally made for unconscious or paralyzed residents who have a hard time keeping the thumb in correct position.
  *(B) This positions a hand in normal alignment and prevents contractures of the thumb and fingers.
    (C) A sling supports the upper extremity; it does not position the fingers in correct alignment.
    (D) This hand does not need to be restrained; it needs to be placed in a normal body position.

22. (A) Giving an opinion makes a judgment that may be different than the resident's values or feelings; the opinion could be a barrier to further communication.
    (B) This limits the chance for the resident to talk about a matter of concern; the resident may not feel comfortable talking about this matter with friends.
    (C) Avoiding communication limits the chance for the resident to talk about a concern.
  *(D) This allows residents to explore options without another person's values changing their opinion.

23. (A) A resident with a colostomy can have a regular diet.
    (B) A colostomy does not affect the ability to walk.
    (C) A normal fluid intake of 2,000 to 2,500 cc (ml) is adequate.
  *(D) Hygiene care will take more time because the colostomy opening (stoma) may require special skin care, and the drainage bag may have to be emptied and cleaned.

24. (A) Touch is used to send a message, not to improve understanding the message.
  *(B) This is important to pick up key words and receive a correct message; listening shows interest.
    (C) Although this is important, it does not improve understanding the message.
    (D) Silence alone will not improve understanding; the NA must listen carefully to get the correct message.

25. (A) This is too short a time for the mouth to recover from the heat of cigarette smoke; the reading would be incorrect.
    (B) Same as (A).
    *(C) It takes 15 minutes for the mouth to recover from the heat of the cigarette smoke and return to the resident's body temperature.
    (D) Not necessary; this is too long a time to wait.

26. *(A) Perineal care is a private activity, and action should be taken to reduce embarrassment.
    (B) This action meets the physical needs of the resident.
    (C) Same as (B).
    (D) Same as (B).

27. (A) This is a physiological reaction to pain.
    *(B) Chronic pain is constant, is difficult to control, and often affects a person's life-style; pain and lack of control can result in the emotional (psychological) response of depression.
    (C) Same as (A).
    (D) Same as (A).

28. *(A) Unsafe; an unconscious resident may react to mouth care by biting down.
    (B) This is a safe tool that can be used to clean the mouth.
    (C) Same as (B).
    (D) Same as (B).

29. (A) This would not provide a written record about the resident's care.
    (B) An NA assignment sheet is made out by the nurse, not the NA.
    *(C) This provides a written record of what should be done for the resident; it promotes communication among staff on different shifts.
    (D) This is not necessary.

30. (A) This reduces anxiety and encourages resident cooperation.
    (B) This should be done because it is expensive to replace personal items such as false teeth, hearing aids, and glasses.
    (C) This provides privacy during the linen change.
    *(D) These linens are considered contaminated and soiled and should never be returned because they will contaminate the linen room.

31. (A) If a gait belt is not used, the resident should be held under the arms and around the shoulder blades.
    *(B) This allows the NA to hold onto the resident firmly and use good body mechanics.
    (C) Not necessary; a weak resident can be transferred safely.
    (D) Unsafe; the resident must be supported by the NA during the transfer.

32. *(A) The NA must first locate the fire to determine how close it is and if the unit is in danger.
   (B) A person cannot take an extinguisher to the fire scene if the location of the fire is not known.
   (C) Unsafe; the first action should be to locate the fire to determine if residents need to be moved.
   (D) This would cause unnecessary confusion; the alarm should only be pulled when the fire is first found.

33. (A) This is a command and challenges the resident.
   (B) This is a command and challenges the resident; when agitated, a person may not be able to control behavior when told.
   (C) He will not be able to sit still when he is agitated; also, it is judgmental.
   *(D) Walking removes the resident from the situation and helps to reduce extra energy; it does not confront the resident.

34. (A) Hot liquids do not prevent chills.
   *(B) This action limits water drying on the skin (evaporation), which prevents a chill.
   (C) This action does not prevent chilling; it increases blood return to the heart.
   (D) Heat lamps are used for treating wounds and require a doctor's order.

35. (A) This needs a signed consent and is only done if nothing else works.
   (B) The hair must be free of tangles before braiding.
   *(C) This limits the amount of hair being combed at a time, which limits discomfort.
   (D) A large-toothed comb should be used; a small-toothed comb is used to remove the head lice eggs (nits) from the hair.

36. (A) The microorganisms on the NA's fingers would contaminate the food.
   *(B) Exposure to the air cools the food and avoids mucous membrane burns due to hot food.
   (C) Foods should be served separately so they retain their own taste and texture.
   (D) The microorganisms in the NA's mouth would contaminate the food.

37. *(A) This would increase feelings of self-worth.
   (B) This is punishment; although rewards should be decided upon by the nurse and resident, praise is always an acceptable reward.
   (C) Residents should never be ignored; all behavior should be addressed in a nonjudgmental way.
   (D) Cigarettes are not good for health, and smoking should not be encouraged by the NA.

38. (A) This is 0.8° F too low.
  *(B) This is the correct measurement; each line on the scale is 0.2 points; two lines above 101 is 101.4° F.
   (C) This is .8° F too high.
   (D) This is 1.2° F too high.

39. *(A) This is a major responsibility of NAs for which they are trained.
   (B) This is part of the legal role of the nurse, not the NA.
   (C) Same as (B).
   (D) Same as (B).

40. *(A) Changing the plan of care is the role of the nurse, not the NA.
   (B) Unsafe; this increases the need for oxygen; respirations will increase and the resident will be short of breath; the resident may also become upset by being rushed; the nurse must change the plan of care; the nurse must change the plan of care.
   (C) Residents need a complete bath at least once a week and whenever necessary; skipping part of the bath does not address the oxygen problem; the nurse must alter the plan of care.
   (D) The nurse must be notified; the plan must be changed because it leaves the resident short of breath; the resident's respiratory needs must be met.

41. (A) This can cut off circulation; it should be snug, not tight.
   (B) This could cause an injury if the rails are lowered while the straps are still tied to the rails.
  *(C) This protects the skin from injury caused by rubbing or pressure.
   (D) Restraints should be released every two hours.

42. *(A) Appropriate; touch says much more than words and it expresses caring and comfort.
   (B) This does not recognize her feelings and is false reassurance.
   (C) This leaves the resident alone when she may already feel alone; by staying the NA gives the resident a chance to talk.
   (D) This does not recognize the resident's feelings; this may not be true.

43. (A) Antibiotics are usually given to treat infection, not prevent infection; this is not the NA's role; it is the nurse's role to teach about medications.
   (B) This would prevent falls, not infection.
  *(C) A resident should wash the hands after toileting to remove microorganisms.
   (D) This can contaminate the urinary meatus and vagina; washing from front to back moves soiled material from clean areas to dirty areas.

44. (A) The feet must be washed before applying lotion.
    (B) Standing in a shower is not as effective as soaking the feet in soap and water.
    (C) Wiping is not as effective as soaking; soap and warm water are needed to clean the feet.
  *(D) Soaking with soap and water allows the skin to be softened and ground-in dirt to be removed.

45. (A) This is active ROM and is performed by the resident.
    (B) This would not move the joints through their full ROM.
  *(C) ROM is passive when another person moves the resident's joints through their full range.
    (D) These were not the instructions on the NA's assignment sheet; ROM is within the NA's job description.

46. (A) Not directly related to nutrition; this measures the pressure of blood in an artery.
  *(B) If nutrition is not adequate, the resident will lose weight.
    (C) This measures air going in and out of the lungs, not level of nutrition.
    (D) This measures the heart rate, not level of nutrition.

47. *(A) Simple words and sentences are more easily understood by confused residents.
    (B) A confused resident may not be able to make a decision.
    (C) This may not be understood by the confused resident.
    (D) This is a threat and should be avoided when talking with residents.

48. (A) This could harm the resident; it could cause muscle strain and bones to fracture.
    (B) Keeping the resident in the Geri-chair could cause muscle strain and bones to fracture.
  *(C) This provides for physical safety and prevents injury by allowing free movement.
    (D) This would be done after the seizure is over.

49. *(A) This answers the question and meets the resident's right to know who is giving care.
    (B) This denies the resident's feelings; residents who are aware of their memory loss are usually upset by this loss.
    (C) This does not answer the resident's question and may make the resident feel guilty.
    (D) No response would make the resident more upset; the resident has a right to know who is giving care.

50. (A) This denies the resident's feelings and may further increase anxiety.
    *(B) This reduces the cause of the anxiety.
     (C) The resident would still be dangling high in the air, which would not reduce anxiety.
     (D) Same as (A).

51. (A) This does not rest the heart; vital signs should be taken after the resident's activity is stopped.
     (B) This only makes the pain worse because activity increases the work of the heart.
    *(C) Decreased activity limits the oxygen demands on the heart, which reduces pain.
     (D) Same as (A).

52. (A) The NA needs more information before reporting to the nurse; the resident may only be in a deep sleep.
     (B) The care giver should first get the resident's attention before giving a direction.
    *(C) Together, touch and using the person's name are the best way to get a response from a resident.
     (D) This would only repeat talking, and the resident has not responded to talking.

53. (A) This may not be appropriate for all residents; a bladder training program must be based on individual needs.
    *(B) All residents, regardless of the specifics of their own program, are toileted upon awakening in the morning.
     (C) Same as (A).
     (D) Same as (A).

54. (A) Not necessary; restraints are only necessary if the resident may harm himself/herself or others.
     (B) Bedrails would be enough to provide for safety.
     (C) Same as (A).
    *(D) This is unsafe; the nurse must decide if the resident needs teaching about safety or is too confused and needs restraints ordered.

55. *(A) Pumping up the cuff too soon would trap blood in the arm, causing an incorrect reading; it would also be painful.
     (B) The blood pressure was not heard because the cuff was released too fast.
     (C) This should have been done before the cuff was pumped up.
     (D) This should be done before and after use.

TEST DRILL 2

Answer Key

1.	C	29.	C
2.	B	30.	D
3.	A	31.	B
4.	A	32.	A
5.	C	33.	D
6.	A	34.	B
7.	B	35.	C
8.	D	36.	B
9.	C	37.	A
10.	D	38.	B
11.	D	39.	A
12.	C	40.	D
13.	A	41.	C
14.	C	42.	A
15.	A	43.	C
16.	D	44.	D
17.	C	45.	C
18.	A	46.	B
19.	C	47.	A
20.	B	48.	C
21.	B	49.	A
22.	D	50.	B
23.	D	51.	C
24.	B	52.	C
25.	C	53.	B
26.	A	54.	D
27.	B	55.	A
28.	A		

TEST DRILL 3

Questions

1. What should the NA do for all types of isolation?
   (A) Wear a gown.
   (B) Keep visitors out.
   (C) Wash the hands.
   (D) Double bag garbage.

2. Mr. Smith is on complete bed rest and needs a complete change of linen. What should the NA do?
   (A) Make an occupied bed.
   (B) Put padding under Mr. Smith.
   (C) Change the draw sheet.
   (D) Have Mr. Smith sit in a chair.

3. Mrs. Cook has a hard time speaking because of a stroke. To increase the resident's ability to communicate her needs, what should the NA do?
   (A) Talk to her, but do not encourage a response.
   (B) Use questions that require yes or no responses.
   (C) Anticipate all her needs to reduce communication.
   (D) Use written or nonverbal gestures to communicate.

4. A resident with a wrist restraint should have the restraint released every:
   (A) 15 minutes.
   (B) 30 minutes.
   (C) 1 hour.
   (D) 2 hours.

5. Mrs. Chase is paranoid and does not like anyone to go into her closet. When returning clean laundry, what should the NA do?
   (A) Put her clothes away when she is out of the room.
   (B) Tell her it is a rule for staff to put clothes away.
   (C) Reassure her that nothing of hers will be taken.
   (D) Allow the resident to put away her own clothes.

6. What should the NA do when the electrical cord on a resident's radio is torn near the plug?
   (A) Wrap it with electrical tape immediately.
   (B) Report it to the nurse at the change of shift.
   (C) Remove the radio and give it to the nurse.
   (D) Unplug it and leave it for a family member.

7. The NA sees another care giver treat a resident in an abusive and abrupt way. What should the NA do?

(A) Reassure the resident.
(B) Report it to the nurse.
(C) Avoid the other care giver.
(D) Talk to the care giver.

8. Mr. Grant is depressed. He states, "When I have the chance, I am going to commit suicide." What should the NA say?

(A) "Don't say that, it's not so bad."
(B) "You have five grandchildren to live for."
(C) "Tell me more about your plans."
(D) "I'll get the nurse to give you some medication."

9. The NA must care for the skin of a resident who is incontinent of urine and stool. To *best* protect the skin, what should the NA apply?

(A) Vaseline-type jelly
(B) Baby powder
(C) Corn starch
(D) A colostomy pouch

10. Where should soiled linen be placed after it is removed from a bed?

(A) On the overbed table
(B) On the floor under the bed
(C) In a soiled linen hamper
(D) Into the linen chute

11. When giving a bed bath, what part of the body should the NA wash *first*?

(A) Axilla
(B) Face
(C) Rectum
(D) Legs

12. To prevent injury when applying a restraint, what should the NA do *first*?

(A) Place the resident in body alignment.
(B) Leave the restraint very loose.
(C) Tie the strap in a double knot.
(D) Pad the bony areas with sheepskin.

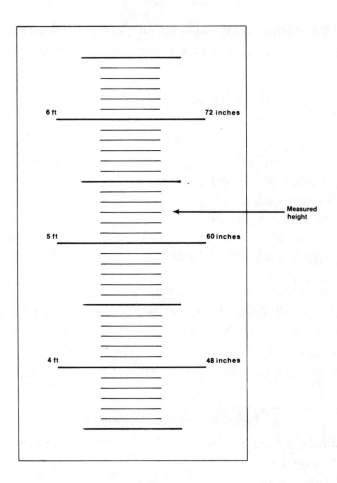

13. The NA measured the height of a resident. Using the drawing above, what is the resident's height?

    (A) 60 inches
    (B) 5½ feet
    (C) 5 feet, 3 inches
    (D) 4 feet, 13 inches

14. When caring for dentures, what should the NA do?

    (A) Store them dry in a denture cup.
    (B) Floss between the teeth of the dentures.
    (C) Rinse the dentures and mouth with mouthwash.
    (D) Brush them at least twice a day.

15. The resident is incontinent during the night. What should the NA say when changing his pajamas?

    (A) Say nothing because it may upset him further.
    (B) "I'm going to change your pajamas now, grandpa."
    (C) "Hello sweetie, I'm going to give you a new set of pajamas."
    (D) "I'm Alice Jones, your NA. I'm going to change your pajamas."

16. A resident has a decubitus at the base of the spine (sacral decubitus). In which of the following positions should the NA place the resident to reduce pressure to the sacral area?

    (A) High Fowler's (high-sitting)
    (B) Supine (back-lying)
    (C) Lateral (side-lying)
    (D) Fowler's (semi-sitting)

17. The NA is to give a back massage to an elderly resident. The skin looks dry, thin, and fragile. What should the NA do?

    (A) Use body lotion.
    (B) Wash with soap.
    (C) Massage with alcohol.
    (D) Use firm, rubbing strokes.

18. A resident who is confused and unsteady when walking has to go to the bathroom. What should the NA do to make the resident safe?

    (A) Encourage her to use the bedpan.
    (B) Stay with her while she is in the bathroom.
    (C) Restrain her to the toilet for safety.
    (D) Keep the bathroom door open and observe her.

19. To meet the legal rules for documentation, how should the NA show that assigned care was given?

    (A) Tell the nurse what was done.
    (B) Record care on the correct NA forms.
    (C) Tell the oncoming NA what was done.
    (D) Keep a diary of the care given.

20. A resident on a bladder retraining program is incontinent at 1 AM every morning. What should the NA do?

    (A) Apply a disposable incontinence pad at bedtime.
    (B) Limit the intake of fluid after the evening meal.
    (C) Leave the call bell within easy reach.
    (D) Wake the resident and toilet before 1 AM.

21. Which of the following is NOT a correct action when taking a blood pressure (BP) reading?

    (A) Tell the BP result if asked by the resident.
    (B) Have the pressure drop by 10 mm Hg per second.
    (C) Support the arm under the wrist and elbow.
    (D) Use a different arm each time the BP is taken.

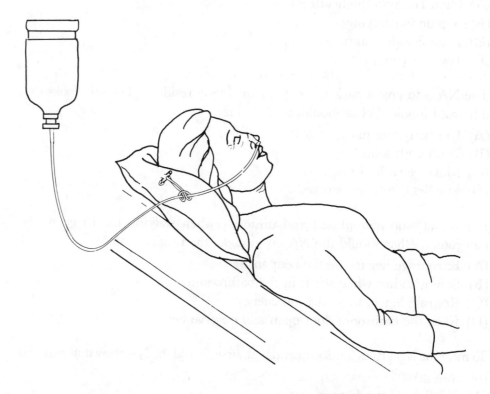

22. The picture above shows equipment that is used to:
    (A) Provide food.
    (B) Deliver oxygen.
    (C) Collect waste.
    (D) Suction mucus.

23. Which of the following would indicate to the NA that a resident was having difficulty breathing?
    (A) Respirations that are 16 per minute and deep
    (B) Respirations that are 18 per minute with resident mouth breathing
    (C) Respirations that are 20 per minute and shallow
    (D) Respirations that are 30 per minute and noisy

24. Mrs. Rack is afraid of falling and gets upset when it is time to get out of bed. To reduce her anxiety, what is the *best* thing the NA should do?
    (A) Allow her to transfer without rushing.
    (B) Make the move easier by using a mechanical lift.
    (C) Explain that there is nothing to worry about.
    (D) Permit her to stay in bed as long as possible.

25. Which of the following residents would require a rectal temperature instead of an oral temperature?

    (A) A man with no teeth
    (B) A resident getting oxygen by mask
    (C) An elderly person with dentures
    (D) A woman who is mentally alert

26. To give safe perineal care to a woman, what should the NA do?

    (A) Apply antiodor spray.
    (B) Avoid using soap in this area.
    (C) Wash from the pubis toward the rectum.
    (D) Dry from the back to the front.

27. Which of the following actions by the NA would support confidentiality and privacy?

    (A) Sharing informaton about a resident during report
    (B) Talking about another resident in front of visitors
    (C) Telling your family about a resident's feelings
    (D) Talking about a resident's diagnosis with a roommate

28. A resident has wrist restraints. What should the NA do to provide an adequate fluid intake?

    (A) Provide a straw to assist with drinking.
    (B) Encourage at least eight ounces of fluid at each meal.
    (C) Place a pitcher of water and glass within reach
    (D) Offer fluids frequently between meals.

29. What is the first step in good communication with a resident?

    (A) Teaching about self-care
    (B) Listening carefully
    (C) Sharing things about yourself
    (D) Talking about happy things

30. Which of the following would be within the normal range for the pulse rate in an elderly resident?

    (A) 30 to 50 beats per minute
    (B) 60 to 100 beats per minute
    (C) 120 to 130 beats per minute
    (D) 140 to 200 beats per minute

31. While eating, Mr. Spot grabs his throat with his hands, appears unable to breathe, and looks very scared. What conclusion should be made by the NA?

    (A) He does not like the food.
    (B) He swallowed a large piece of meat.
    (C) He has food caught in his airway.
    (D) He ate food that is too hot.

32. What should the NA do to provide for resident safety while making an occupied bed?

   (A) Remove the pillow while the bed is being made.
   (B) Keep the side rail up on the working side of the bed.
   (C) Tell the resident to use the call bell for help.
   (D) Check for any tubing coming from the resident.

33. A resident who needs more supervision is moved to a room closer to the nurse's station. The resident is very anxious. What should the NA do?

   (A) Tell her she will meet new friends.
   (B) Keep her as active as possible during the day.
   (C) Encourage the resident to share her feelings.
   (D) Focus on something other than her anxiety.

34. The resident is dying and is sad and depressed. What should the NA do?

   (A) Try to cheer him up.
   (B) Explain that he still has time to live.
   (C) Accept his anger as a healthy response.
   (D) Listen to his concerns about leaving his family.

35. To check for blueness due to lack of oxygen (cyanosis), in what area should the NA look?

   (A) The buttocks
   (B) The whites of both eyes
   (C) The fingernail beds
   (D) The area around the wrists

36. Mrs. Zeider has an above-the-elbow amputation. She tells the NA that she prefers to be sitting in a chair to put on the false arm (prosthesis). What should the NA do?

   (A) Tell her that it is safer to put it on while in bed.
   (B) Explain that she must put the prosthesis on in bed.
   (C) Tell the nurse so it can be added to the nursing care plan.
   (D) Put the prosthesis on when she is sitting on the side of the bed.

37. What should the NA do when finding a resident on the floor after a fall?

   (A) Move the resident back to bed.
   (B) Call the nurse to assess the resident.
   (C) Sit the resident in a chair.
   (D) See if the resident can stand.

38. What should NAs do to avoid unpleasant mouth odor in their own mouths?

   (A) Brush the teeth after meals.
   (B) Use deodorant daily.
   (C) Rinse with salt water.
   (D) Avoid alcoholic drinks.

39. Which of the following should the NA immediately report to the nurse?
    (A) Dandruff
    (B) Head lice
    (C) Dirty hair
    (D) Matted hair

40. To protect the confused resident at night, which of the following should the NA do first?
    (A) Raise both of the side rails.
    (B) Leave on a small light.
    (C) Place a urinal/bedpan in the bed.
    (D) Check on the resident often.

41. Which of the following would NOT limit the spread of microorganisms?
    (A) Wearing a clean uniform
    (B) Cleaning shoes
    (C) Wearing perfume
    (D) Washing the hair

42. Mrs. Pits enjoys the visits of animals provided by a local animal shelter. After one of these visits, Mrs. Pits sadly tells the NA about a dog she onced owned. What should the NA do?
    (A) Arrange for more frequent vists by the animal shelter.
    (B) Ask Mrs. Pits to tell more about her dog.
    (C) Get her a book about animals out of the library.
    (D) Share with Mrs. Pits a story about a pet.

43. When a resident is on bed rest, what is the best exercise that can be done?
    (A) Passive range of motion (ROM)
    (B) Active-assistive exercises
    (C) Contracting and relaxing muscles
    (D) Active range of motion

44. Which of the following is a responsibility of the NA?
    (A) Changing sterile dressings
    (B) Helping nurses with giving out medications
    (C) Assisting residents with grooming
    (D) Writing nursing care plans

45. The NA is measuring the height and weight of a newly admitted resident. When the resident is told her height, she says, "That is one inch shorter than I was 20 years ago." What should the NA do?
    (A) Recognize that this is part of normal aging.
    (B) Explain that people do not usually get shorter.
    (C) Report the resident's loss in height immediately.
    (D) Tell her that it could be the sign of a problem.

46. Mrs. Jones dies and the NA begins postmortem care. Which of the following should the NA do?

    (A) Remove all jewelry.
    (B) Remove the dentures carefully.
    (C) Close the eyes gently.
    (D) Raise the head of the bed slightly.

47. Which of the following will prevent injury to the feet?

    (A) Visiting the podiatrist monthly
    (B) Wearing well-fitted shoes
    (C) Raising the feet when possible
    (D) Wearing cotton socks to sleep

48. When a resident has a urinary tube (Foley) to drain urine from the bladder, the collection bag should be:

    (A) Kept below the level of the bladder.
    (B) Disconnected and rinsed with water every day.
    (C) Placed on the bedrail at the level of the heart.
    (D) Emptied and measured once a day.

49. Mrs. Adams is in constant pain from arthritis and does not like to be touched. What should the NA do?

    (A) Reassure her that she will not feel pain during care.
    (B) Perform care quickly first thing in the morning.
    (C) Let her care for herself and do not touch her.
    (D) Touch her gently when giving necessary care.

50. Mrs. Golden has a history of heart disease. Right after she walks back from lunch she sits in a chair, holds her hand against her chest, and complains of a severe upset stomach. The NA should:

    (A) Listen to her complaints.
    (B) Call the nurse immediately.
    (C) Sit with her quietly.
    (D) Ask the nurse for an antacid.

51. Which of the following actions by the NA would help meet a resident's basic need for security and safety?

    (A) Calling the resident by name
    (B) Making sure that the resident receives enough fluid
    (C) Explaining what is going to be done and why
    (D) Hugging and showing love

52.Which of the following is NOT used to prevent a decubitus?

(A) Sheepskin
(B) Eggcrate mattress
(C) Water mattress
(D) Walker

53. Mrs. West was admitted to the nursing home last week. While the NA was giving care, the resident said, ''I feel that nobody cares about me.'' What should the NA say?

(A) ''That's not true, your daughter loves you.''
(B) ''We all love you here.''
(C) ''Are you angry at your family?''
(D) ''You feel as though nobody cares?''

54. Of the following, what is the safest way to identify a resident?

(A) Telling him to state his full name
(B) Calling him by name and watching his response
(C) Looking at the name on the bed
(D) Checking the identification bracelet

55. A resident with slight left-side weakness needs to be transferred. To best provide for the resident's safety while transferring, where should the NA stand?

(A) Behind the resident
(B) On the resident's left side
(C) In front of the resident
(D) On the resident's right side

TEST DRILL 3

Reasons for Answers

The asterisk (*) is in front of the correct answer.

1. (A) A gown is only worn if direct resident care is given or if the resident is on strict isolation.
    (B) Visitors are allowed after they are told what they must do to maintain isolation.
    *(C) This is done before going into the room or leaving the room for all types of isolation.
    (D) This is unnecessary for protective (reverse) isolation.

2. *(A) An occupied bed is made when a person is on complete bed rest and not allowed out of bed.
    (B) Inadequate; the whole bed must be changed.
    (C) Same as (B).
    (D) Unsafe; the resident is not allowed out of bed.

3. (A) The resident should be involved; communication is a two-way process.
    *(B) Includes the resident and keeps the response simple.
    (C) Same as (A).
    (D) Unnecessary; the resident has a problem with speaking, not hearing.

4. (A) This is the time frame for checking for circulation not restraint release.
    (B) Unnecessary; it only has to be released every 2 hours.
    (C) Same as (B).
    *(D) This is how often a restraint should be released and the area massaged and exercised.

5. (A) This would only add to her paranoia because she would know someone had been in her closet.
    (B) This may not be the policy; the NA would still be in control; the resident needs control.
    (C) Paranoia is not reduced by logic; also false reassurance because sometimes things are lost.
    *(D) This gives the resident control of her personal space.

6. (A) Unsafe; electrical equipment must be repaired by a trained person.
    (B) Unsafe; it should be removed immediately.
    *(C) This action removes it from use and allows the nurse to arrange repair.
    (D) Unsafe; it should be removed from the bedside.

7. (A) This will not stop the behavior of the care giver.
   *(B) Abusive acts are not legally, morally, or ethically right; the nurse has the responsibility and power to stop the abusive acts.
   (C) Same as (A).
   (D) This is not the job of the NA; it should be reported to the nurse in charge.

8. (A) This ignores feelings; false reassurance.
   (B) This ignores feelings and may make him feel guilty about his feelings.
   *(C) Encourages communication; if the resident has specific plans, the threat of suicide is real.
   (D) Ignores feelings; the resident needs to talk about feelings, not run away from them; this statement may be a cry for both physical and emotional help.

9. *(A) Ointments/jellies hold moisture and prevent drying and cracking; the oil base provides a barrier.
   (B) When mixed with moisture, it can cake on the skin and promote the growth of microorganisms.
   (C) Same as (B).
   (D) This should only be placed around an opening in the abdominal wall (stoma) for collection of waste from the body.

10. (A) Soiled linen contaminates furniture.
    (B) Soiled linen contaminates the floor; in most cases the floor is already heavily contaminated and the NA will become exposed to more microorganisms when picking up the linen.
    *(C) This is the safest way to contain soiled linen and microorganisms.
    (D) Linen should be bagged before being put in a linen chute; many facilities do not have laundry chutes.

11. (A) This area is moist and has many microorganisms and should be washed after the face.
    *(B) Most baths are done starting with the face and going toward the feet; bathing should move from clean areas to dirty areas.
    (C) This area is done later in the bath; bathing should move from clean areas to dirty areas.
    (D) Same as (C).

12. *(A) This keeps muscles, joints, and bones in natural position, reducing stress on body parts.
    (B) Restraints must be snug to provide security, yet loose enough for some movement.
    (C) This should only be tied in a slipknot for easy release in an emergency.
    (D) Important, but good body alignment comes first.

13. (A) Three inches too short; 60 inches is equal to 5 feet.
    (B) Three inches too long; 5½ feet is equal to 66 inches.
  *(C) Correct measurement; 5 feet, 3 inches is equal to 63 inches; each line on the scale is equal to 1 inch.
    (D) Two inches too short; inaccurate way to record height; 4 feet, 13 inches should be recorded as 5 feet, 1 inch.

14. (A) Dentures must be stored in water or they will dry out and change shape.
    (B) Not necessary with dentures; flossing removes plaque and tartar between normal teeth that cause gum disease and decay.
    (C) Rinsing with mouthwash is not as thorough as brushing.
  *(D) All surfaces of dentures should be brushed to remove debris at least twice a day and whenever necessary.

15. (A) What happened should not be ignored; the resident has a right to know who is giving care and what will be done.
    (B) An undignified response; he has a right to be called by his own name, which is a sign of respect.
    (C) The resident has a right to be called by his own name; giving him pajamas is not enough; he may need help with changing.
  *(D) This meets the resident's right to know who is giving care and what will be done.

16. (A) In this position body weight is placed on the buttocks and sacrum; the area is exposed to pressure and shearing force.
    (B) In this position the sacrum bears the body's weight, which causes pressure.
  *(C) In this position the hips and side of the body bear the body's weight; this applies no pressure to the sacrum.
    (D) Same as (A).

17. *(A) This reduces friction of the hands against the skin and prevents injury to the skin.
    (B) This should be avoided because it can further dry the skin.
    (C) Same as (B).
    (D) This can cause skin tears and injury to delicate, thin skin; light strokes should be used.

18. (A) Unnecessary; residents should toilet as normally as possible.
  *(B) Confused and unsteady residents must always be assisted in the bathroom to provide for safety.
    (C) Unsafe; residents cannot be safely restrained to a toilet.
    (D) Bathroom doors should be closed for privacy.

19. (A) Although this would be done, it is not written proof that care was given and does not meet legal requirements for documentation.

   *(B) Recording care given provides a written legal record of the care received by the resident.

   (C) Same as (A).

   (D) This is not a legal record.

20. (A) This keeps the skin moist, which can cause skin breakdown.

   (B) This might decrease the amount voided but may not prevent incontinence.

   (C) The resident may not be aware of the need to void before it is too late to call for help.

   *(D) This allows the resident the chance to void before becoming incontinent.

21. (A) The resident has the right to know the reading.

   *(B) The pressure should drop by 2 to 3 mm Hg per second.

   (C) This promotes a correct reading; if not supported, the reading could be abnormally high.

   (D) The results would not be consistent; the same arm should be used.

22. *(A) This is a nasogastric tube, which goes into the nose, down the esophagus, and into the stomach; fluids can be passed through the tube to feed a person.

   (B) This is a double-pronged tube in the nose that delivers oxygen (nasal cannula); this tube is attached to wall oxygen or to a tank of oxygen, not a tube feeding bag that is shown in the drawing.

   (C) A urinary tube (Foley) goes into the urinary bladder and drains urine; the drawing is of a tube feeding.

   (D) The nurse may put a small tube into a person's mouth or nose for several seconds to remove clogged mucus; the drawing is of a tube feeding.

23. (A) These are within normal limits.

   (B) This rate is within normal limits; mouth breathing can be a habit and does not indicate respiratory distress.

   (C) Same as (A).

   *(D) This person may be in respiratory distress; this rate is outside the normal range of 14 to 20 respirations per minute; normal respirations are usually noiseless.

24. *(A) This gives her control by allowing her to set the pace of the transfer; the ability to control a situation usually reduces anxiety.

   (B) This would make the resident feel more dependent, helpless, and out of control.

   (C) This is false reassurance and will not reduce her fear.

   (D) This would not decrease anxiety; the waiting and thinking about the transfer could increase anxiety.

25. (A) An accurate oral reading can be obtained.
    *(B) Oral reading unsafe; an oral temperature of a person receiving oxygen
         by mask would be abnormally low; to take the temperature the NA would
         have to remove the oxygen mask, which would limit the oxygen intake
         of the resident.
     (C) Same as (A).
     (D) Same as (A).

26. (A) This should be avoided; it can be irritating and cause a rash.
     (B) Soap and water are most effective when washing the perineal area.
    *(C) This moves soiled material away from the urinary meatus and vagina
         toward the rectum, thereby reducing the chance of a urinary tract infection.
     (D) This should be avoided because it would be moving stool from a dirty
         area (rectum) toward a cleaner area (pubis).

27. *(A) This is correct behavior; the purpose of report is to share and communicate
         important information about residents.
     (B) This action fails to support confidentiality; information can only be shared
         with health team members.
     (C) Same as (B).
     (D) Same as (B).

28. (A) While a straw can assist drinking, this answer does address encourage-
         ment of fluid intake.
     (B) An intake of 720 cc (ml) is not adequate; 2,000 to 2,500 cc (ml) daily is
         required to maintain normal fluid volume.
     (C) This is useless when the resident's wrists are restrained.
    *(D) Because of restrained wrists the resident must depend on the NA to pro-
         vide fluids.

29. (A) Listening comes before teaching.
    *(B) A message must be heard before an NA can respond.
     (C) The focus of communication should be on residents and their needs.
     (D) Sometimes residents have a need to talk about sad topics such as death
         and dying; these talks can be meaningful and helpful.

30. (A) This range is too low.
    *(B) This is the normal range for a pulse in an elderly person.
     (C) This range is too high.
     (D) Same as (C).

31. (A) This is not a likely reaction if he was unhappy with the food.
     (B) Swallowing a large piece of food will not obstruct breathing.
    *(C) Grabbing the throat is a common universal (classic) sign of airway obstruc-
         tion; not being able to breathe and the resulting fear are signs of a blocked
         airway.
     (D) The usual response to hot food is to spit it out of the mouth.

32. (A) The pillow should be in place at all times to provide support for the resident's head and neck and should only be removed when changing the pillowcase.
    (B) Unnecessary; the rail needs to be up on the nonworking side.
    (C) Unnecessary; the NA will already be at the bedside.
  *(D) This alerts the NA to the presence of tubes; care should be taken to avoid pulling out a tube when changing the linen.

33. (A) This ignores her feelings; could be false reassurance.
    (B) This ignores her feelings; new activities could increase anxiety.
  *(C) Talking about the change helps to explore feelings, limit tension, and reduce anxiety.
    (D) This ignores her feelings; avoiding what is bothering her could increase anxiety.

34. (A) This is inappropriate; it denies the resident's feelings.
    (B) This ignores his feelings.
    (C) The resident is sad and depressed, not angry; anger is the 2nd stage of dying, while sadness is the 4th stage.
  *(D) The resident needs someone to listen; according to Dr. Kubler-Ross, a leading researcher in death and dying, depression is the 4th stage of dying; people may cry, say little or mourn people who will be left behind.

35. (A) This is where you would look for redness related to pressure, not cyanosis.
    (B) This area is checked for yellow coloring (jaundice), which usually occurs with problems of the liver.
  *(C) This area often turns blue from lack of oxygen because it is far from the heart.
    (D) This area is unrelated to cyanosis due to lack of oxygen.

36. (A) Not always true; this ignores her choice to put it on while sitting in a chair.
    (B) Residents have a right to choose when to put on such things as a prosthesis.
  *(C) This permits more consistent care because her choice is communicated to other health team members.
    (D) This is not her choice; she should be allowed to put it on while sitting in a chair.

37. (A) Moving an injured person could make the injury worse.
  *(B) A trained person must determine if a splint is necessary before moving a resident who has fallen.
    (C) Same as (A).
    (D) Same as (A).

38. *(A) This removes particles of food and debris from the teeth and mouth that can cause mouth odors.
    (B) This is used for the underarms.
    (C) This might wash out some food particles but would not remove the debris between the teeth.
    (D) Alcohol should never be consumed before or during work.

39. (A) Although this should be reported, it is not an emergency.
    *(B) Head lice can spread directly and indirectly to others; the resident must be isolated until the hair is treated and the room and belongings are disinfected.
    (C) Same as (A).
    (D) Not necessary; grooming is within the NA job description.

40. *(A) Rails provide a barrier and help to remind residents that they are in bed.
    (B) This would not provide a barrier to prevent falls, although a small light could help limit confusion.
    (C) This would not provide a barrier to prevent falls; although this would reduce the need to get out of bed, it could make the person feel uncomfortable.
    (D) This would not provide a barrier to prevent falls.

41. (A) This limits microorganisms on the clothes.
    (B) The ground and floor are considered dirty (contaminated) and shoes should be cleaned often.
    *(C) This is not related to infection control.
    (D) This limits microorganisms on the hair.

42. (A) This would not meet the resident's present need to talk about the past; this could also be impractical or impossible.
    *(B) This encourages the resident to talk about past happy times.
    (C) This would not meet the resident's present need to talk; reading is not a shared activity.
    (D) This focuses on the NA rather than the resident and should be avoided.

43. (A) This increases joint mobility and circulation but does little for muscle tone.
    (B) The resident who is able should do active ROM without assistance.
    (C) This is isometric exercise; it increases muscle tone but does not move joints.
    *(D) This requires the resident to move joints and muscles through full ROM and is called isotonic exercise; it increases joint mobility, circulation, and muscle tone.

44. (A) This is not part of the NA job description; sterile dressings are done by the nurse.
    (B) It is illegal for an NA to administer medication.
    *(C) This is one of the main roles of the NA.
    (D) This is not part of the NA job description; it is the role of the nurse; the NA can contribute information but cannot write on the nursing care plan.

45. *(A) People get slightly shorter as the musculoskeletal and nervous systems change with aging.
    (B) This is incorrect information; people can get slightly shorter as the musculoskeletal and nervous systems change with aging.
    (C) This is not an emergency, it is part of the normal aging process.
    (D) This would upset the resident; it is part of the normal aging process.

46. (A) The wedding band should be left on and taped to the body.
    (B) Dentures should be placed back into the mouth.
    *(C) The body should be placed in natural alignment because it is difficult to reposition the body after rigor mortis sets in.
    (D) Same as (C).

47. (A) Podiatrists prevent or treat problems but do not prevent injury.
    *(B) This prevents many skin problems such as blisters, corns, decubiti of the feet, and abrasions.
    (C) This reduces swelling (edema); this does not prevent injury.
    (D) This helps keep the feet dry but does not prevent injury.

48. *(A) This allows urine to drain by gravity and not flow back into the bladder.
    (B) A urine drainage system should not be opened; this prevents micro-organisms from causing a urinary tract infection.
    (C) This would not allow urine to drain by gravity.
    (D) The drainage bag should be measured more frequently; output is usually measured every eight hours or after each shift.

49. (A) This is false reassurance.
    (B) People in pain need to move slowly; people with arthritis have more stiffness and pain in the morning; when possible care should be given later in the day.
    (C) Some touching is necessary; she is probably unable to give herself total care.
    *(D) Some touching is necessary; being gentle keeps pain to a minimum.

50. (A) Unsafe; she needs immediate help from the nurse.
    *(B) Her pain may be due to a heart problem, and she needs a professional assessment of her condition.
    (C) Same as (A).
    (D) Her pain may be caused by a heart problem rather than a stomach problem; further assessment is needed.

51. (A) This meets a person's need for dignity and self-esteem.
    (B) This meets the basic physiological need for adequate fluids.
    *(C) Not knowing what is going to happen and why can be frightening; explaining what will happen and why will make a person feel more secure.
    (D) This meets the need for love and belonging.

52. (A) This reduces rubbing (friction) and allows air to flow through the tufts of lamb's wool, keeping the skin dry and preventing decubiti.
   (B) This spreads body weight more evenly over the peaks in the mattress, reducing pressure.
   (C) This spreads body weight along the entire mattress, reducing pressure over bony body parts.
  *(D) This does not prevent pressure; promotes balance by widening the base of support.

53. (A) This is false reassurance; it may or may not be true.
   (B) This may not be true and does not address the resident's feelings of being unwanted by the family.
   (C) Direct questions should be avoided; the resident may be hurt or sad, not angry.
  *(D) This is open ended and encourages the resident to talk more about feelings.

54. (A) Not safe; the resident may be confused.
   (B) Same as (A).
   (C) Not safe; the resident may be in the wrong bed.
  *(D) This is the most accurate method of identification; on admission residents usually receive a bracelet with their name.

55. (A) Unsafe; this would place the NA on the other side of the bed.
   (B) Unsafe; when transferring from bed to a chair the resident should lean forward while moving to the standing position; this movement requires the NA to stand in front of the resident to provide support.
  *(C) This provides support when the resident leans forward while moving to a standing position and enables the NA to direct movement toward the chair in a safe manner.
   (D) Same as (B).

TEST DRILL 3

Answer Key

1.	C	29.	B
2.	A	30.	B
3.	B	31.	C
4.	D	32.	D
5.	D	33.	C
6.	C	34.	D
7.	B	35.	C
8.	C	36.	C
9.	A	37.	B
10.	C	38.	A
11.	B	39.	B
12.	A	40.	A
13.	C	41.	C
14.	D	42.	B
15.	D	43.	D
16.	C	44.	C
17.	A	45.	A
18.	B	46.	C
19.	B	47.	B
20.	D	48.	A
21.	B	49.	D
22.	A	50.	B
23.	D	51.	C
24.	A	52.	D
25.	B	53.	D
26.	C	54.	D
27.	A	55.	C
28.	D		

CHAPTER 6

Practice Questions with Reasons for Answers

THE ROLE OF THE NURSE AIDE

This section includes questions related to personal health and safety, values, ethics, legal aspects of nurse aide (NA) practice, documentation and reporting, care planning, the role of the NA and its limitations, and the reporting of resident maltreatment.

Questions

1. The NA is assigned to a resident who transfers to a chair with a mechanical lift. It has been a long time since the NA used the lift. What should the NA do?
   (A) Ask the nurse to demonstrate how to use the lift.
   (B) Keep the resident in bed for the day.
   (C) Ask another NA to explain how to use the lift.
   (D) Use the lift and hope that it works.

2. When the condition of a resident changes, what should the NA do?
   (A) Document the observed changes.
   (B) Report the changes to the nurse.
   (C) Notify the doctor.
   (D) Call the family.

3. Which of the following statements is true about an NA's smoking?
   (A) Smoking is not harmful.
   (B) Smoking can be unpleasant to others.
   (C) Smoking can be done anywhere.
   (D) Smoking is an inexpensive habit.

4. The nurse asks the NA to do something that is outside the legal scope of the NA role. What should the NA do *first*?
   (A) Do the task and file a grievance later.
   (B) Call the supervisor immediately.
   (C) Refuse to do the assigned task.
   (D) Call the union representative.

5. With what is ethics concerned?

   (A) Right or wrong behavior
   (B) A public crime
   (C) A civil law
   (D) Careless actions

6. The nursing care plan directs the NA to assist the resident in a tub bath at 10 AM. However, the resident has just returned from physical therapy, is tired, and refuses the bath. What should the NA do?

   (A) Give a shower instead.
   (B) Cancel the bath.
   (C) Give the tub bath anyway.
   (D) Tell the nurse.

7. An NA finds a resident spreading stool on himself, the linens, and the bedrails. The resident goal that would be most easily met by the NA would be: The resident will:

   (A) Stop spreading stool.
   (B) Be clean and dry.
   (C) Call the NA for the bedpan.
   (D) Toilet himself when needed.

8. A resident weighing 165 pounds is on a reduced calorie diet. The resident's goal is to lose 2 pounds every week. Which of the following weights would meet the goal?

   (A) 167 pounds
   (B) 165 pounds
   (C) 164 pounds
   (D) 163 pounds

9. The NA provides passive range of motion (ROM) to a resident to maintain joint movement. This goal would NOT be met if the resident developed a/an:

   (A) Contracture.
   (B) Decubitus.
   (C) Rash.
   (D) Infection.

10. What is the most important reason why the NA must fully understand how to do a procedure before doing it for a resident?

    (A) To explain the procedure to the resident
    (B) To complete the procedure safely
    (C) To teach a new NA the procedure
    (D) To perform the procedure quickly

11. Which of the following actions is within the NA job description?
    (A) Supervising a new NA on the unit
    (B) Telling residents what is wrong with them
    (C) Observing and reporting unusual symptoms
    (D) Giving medication when directed by the nurse

12. When arriving on duty in the morning, what should the NA do *first*?
    (A) Get a cup of coffee.
    (B) Check the assignment sheet for who gets morning baths.
    (C) Care for independent residents.
    (D) Check the safety of assigned residents.

13. When is the administration of medication by an NA permitted?
    (A) Sometimes
    (B) With meals
    (C) Never
    (D) At night

14. When planning the workday, which of the following is the *most* important activity of the NA?
    (A) Attending staff education programs
    (B) Carrying out direct orders from the doctor
    (C) Completing cleaning duties
    (D) Protecting the safety of residents

Reasons for the answers

The asterisk (*) is in front of the correct answer.

1. *(A) The nurse is the NA's immediate supervisor and the person the NA should turn to for help.
   (B) This would not meet the resident's need to get out of bed or the NA's need to relearn how to use the mechanical lift.
   (C) An NA is not responsible for teaching another NA; the nurse is the correct resource person.
   (D) Unsafe; the resident could get hurt if correct technique is not used.

2. (A) Although important, changes must be immediately brought to the attention of the nurse because emergency care may be necessary.
   *(B) The nurse must respond to changes in the condition of the resident because further assessment or treatment may be necessary.
   (C) This is the responsibility of the nurse.
   (D) This is the responsibility of the nurse or doctor.

3. (A) Smoking has been proved to cause diseases such as lung cancer.
   *(B) Smoke is irritating to the mucous membranes, and second-hand smoke can cause disease in a nonsmoker.
   (C) There are special smoking areas to protect the rights of nonsmokers and to meet fire safety rules.
   (D) Cigarettes are expensive, not inexpensive.

4. (A) NAs should not perform tasks they are not licensed to perform.
   (B) This should be done if the nurse threatens the NA or continues to insist that the task be performed; the first action should be to refuse to do the task.
   *(C) Performing a task that one is not licensed to do is illegal; the NA has the right to refuse to follow an order outside the NA job description.
   (D) Same as (B).

5. *(A) Ethics involves making judgments about how one should act or not act.
   (B) Criminal laws involve bad actions against society.
   (C) Civil laws are concerned with how people interact in a relationship.
   (D) This relates to negligence.

6. (A) Residents have a right to refuse care.
   (B) Although this may be done, it is the nurse who makes this decision.
   (C) Same as (A).
   *(D) The nursing care plan may need to be changed; the nurse responsible for the resident must be told that the resident refused care.

7. (A) The resident's mental condition may prevent him from understanding his actions; this goal may never be achieved.
 *(B) Keeping residents clean and well groomed, which are basic physical needs, are major responsibilities of the NA.
  (C) Same as (A).
  (D) Same as (A).

8. (A) Goal not met; this would be a 2-pound weight gain.
  (B) Goal not met; the weight remained the same.
  (C) Goal not met; 1 pound, not 2 pounds, was lost.
 *(D) The goal was met; this is a 2-pound weight loss.

9. *(A) Contractures should not develop if ROM is correctly done.
  (B) This is related to pressure, not ROM.
  (C) This is not related to ROM.
  (D) Same as (C).

10. (A) While it is important to explain care to residents, safety is the main reason the NA learns how to perform a procedure prior to doing it for a resident.
 *(B) Safety of the resident is always most important; the NA must only perform skills that are within the legal role of the NA, are understood, and have been practiced.
  (C) NAs are trained and supervised by the nurse, not other NAs.
  (D) While this might be desirable, the primary goal is to maintain resident safety when providing care.

11. (A) This is not part of the NA job description; an NA should work under the direct supervision of a nurse.
  (B) This is the role of the doctor; the nurse can reinforce this information.
 *(C) This is part of the NA job description; the NA is trained to identify major abnormal signs and symptoms.
  (D) This is the role of the nurse; it is illegal for the NA to give medications, even if directed by the nurse.

12. (A) The NA should begin work at the start of the shift.
  (B) Bathing schedules may change because they depend on the immediate needs and requests of residents.
  (C) This would ignore dependent residents.
 *(D) This is necessary before morning care can begin.

13. (A) NAs should never give medications to a resident regardless of the situation.
  (B) Same as (A).
 *(C) Nurses, not NAs, are licensed to administer medications; it is illegal for NAs to give a resident medicine.
  (D) Same as (A).

14. (A) Important but only after resident safety is maintained.
    (B) The nurse, not the NA, is responsible for ensuring that doctor's orders are carried out; the NA works under the supervision of the nurse.
    (C) Same as (A).
    *(D) Maintaining resident safety is a major part of the NA job responsibilities.

THE AGING PROCESS AND BASIC HUMAN NEEDS

This section includes questions related to the physical changes of aging, developmental tasks of the older age groups, and basic human needs, which include physiological, security and safety, love, self-esteem, and self-actualization needs.

Questions

1. Which of the following actions by the nurse aide (NA) would help a resident meet a basic physical need?
   (A) Pulling up the side rail after care
   (B) Encouraging a resident to do an activity
   (C) Answering a call light quickly
   (D) Placing a resident back in bed to sleep

2. A resident paints pictures and hangs them in the hall of the nursing home. Which basic human need is being met by this action?
   (A) Love and belonging
   (B) Physiological
   (C) Self-esteem
   (D) Safety and security

3. Which of the following actions would meet a resident's basic physical need?
   (A) Talking with the resident
   (B) Putting up side rails
   (C) Admiring a sweater
   (D) Giving physical hygiene

4. Which of the following is the most basic of the human needs?
   (A) Physiological needs
   (B) Love and belonging needs
   (C) Safety and security needs
   (D) Self-esteem needs

5. A developmental task of the elderly is:
   (A) Helping grown children.
   (B) Preparing for death.
   (C) Developing trust.
   (D) Becoming independent.

6. The growth and development process:
   (A) Follows a pattern.
   (B) Is completed in adulthood.
   (C) Depends on ability.
   (D) Is a simple process.

7. Mr. George has not been sleeping well at night. The NA should:

(A) Take him for a long walk before bedtime.

(B) Ask the nurse to give him a sleeping medication.

(C) Give him a warm cup of tea at bedtime.

(D) Encourage him to be up and active in the daytime.

8. In relation to wellness and illness, how do most older adults see themselves?

(A) As healthy

(B) As sick

(C) As dependent

(D) As helpless

9. What is a word that describes the process of growth and development?

(A) Fast

(B) Individual

(C) Simple

(D) Limiting

10. The rate of the process of growth and development over the life span can be described as:

(A) Uneven.

(B) Complex.

(C) Slow.

(D) Fast.

11. In the elderly, the process of growth and development usually:

(A) Goes backward.

(B) Continues forward.

(C) Becomes more difficult.

(D) Has been completed.

Reasons for the answers

The asterisk (*) is in front of the correct answer.

1.   (A) This supports the need to feel safe and secure.
     (B) This supports the need to feel that one belongs.
     (C) Same as (A).
    *(D) This supports the basic physiological need for sleep.

2.   (A) This relates to closeness, affection, and meaningful relationships.
     (B) This relates to the need for oxygen, food, water, rest, sleep, and elimination.
    *(C) Esteem refers to one's self-worth; if a person's creative works are well liked by others, it supports a person's self-esteem needs.
     (D) This relates to shelter and protection from harm.

3.   (A) This relates to emotional needs.
     (B) This relates to safety needs.
     (C) This relates to self-esteem needs.
    *(D) This is a basic physical need for hygiene.

4. *(A) Physiological needs are basic to life; oxygen, water, food, sleep, and elimination needs must be met before needs on a higher level can be met.
     (B) This is the third basic need.
     (C) This is the second basic need.
     (D) This is the fourth basic need.

5.   (A) This is a developmental task of middle adulthood.
    *(B) The elderly must review their life and face the fact that their deaths are expected.
     (C) This is a developmental task of an infant.
     (D) This is a developmental task during the teenage years.

6. *(A) Although everyone is an individual, the growth and development process follows a general timetable.
     (B) Growth and development continue to the day we die.
     (C) Ability is what emerges from growth and development.
     (D) The growth and development process is complex.

7.   (A) This action would increase circulation and respirations and make a person more awake.
     (B) Sleeping medication should not be used routinely or before other measures are tried first.
     (C) Tea has caffeine, a stimulant, which would keep him awake.
    *(D) Avoiding naps during the day and an active routine should result in a person's being more tired at night.

8. *(A) When asked, most elderly people say they are healthy.
    (B) Older adults measure health by how well they function rather than by the presence of disease; they do not see themselves as ill.
    (C) Most older adults are independent, not dependent.
    (D) Most older adults do not see themselves as helpless because most older adults are independent.

9. (A) Some stages are faster and some are slower depending on the person and the developmental level.
    *(B) Although people follow a general pattern, they do not grow and develop at exactly the same rate or extent.
    (C) The growth and development process is very complex and influenced by many different factors.
    (D) Just the opposite, the growth and development process helps people to extend themselves to be the most that they can be.

10. *(A) The growth and development process occurs in spurts, not at an even pace through the life cycle.
    (B) The process of growth and development is complex, not its rate.
    (C) Although some stages are slower than other stages and some people move through stages more slowly than other people, the growth and development process as a whole is uneven.
    (D) Although some stages are faster than other stages and some people move through stages more quickly than other people, the growth and development process as a whole is uneven.

11. (A) While some older people may act childlike, their process of growth and development is still forward, not backward.
    *(B) The growth and development process is an ongoing one that continues until death.
    (C) The difficulty in dealing with stages of development is related to how the individual *reacts* to the stage rather than the stage itself.
    (D) Same as (B).

PSYCHOSOCIAL NEEDS AND COMMUNICATION

This section includes questions related to residents' rights and meeting emotional, social, and spiritual needs of residents.

Questions

1. Which of the following actions would NOT support a resident's right to privacy?
   (A) Talking about a resident in the lunchroom
   (B) Using a bath blanket during a bath
   (C) Pulling the curtain around a resident using a commode
   (D) Closing the door to the tub room when in use

2. The MOST important thing to teach a newly admitted resident is:
   (A) How to use the call light.
   (B) When meals will be served.
   (C) Why side rails are used.
   (D) Who is in charge of the unit.

3. What should the nurse aide (NA) do first before getting the equipment for a procedure?
   (A) Position the resident for the procedure.
   (B) Pull the resident's curtain around the bed.
   (C) Raise the resident's bed to its highest position.
   (D) Tell the resident what is going to be done.

4. An agitated resident tells the NA that life is no longer worth living and she wants to die. Whom should the NA NOT tell about this statement?
   (A) The resident's doctor
   (B) The social worker
   (C) The resident's roommate
   (D) The charge nurse

5. Which of the following actions by the NA would support confidentiality?
   (A) Avoiding talking about a resident with another resident
   (B) Looking at the chart of an unassigned resident
   (C) Telling others about another resident's wig
   (D) Joking about a resident who has an odor

6. To provide for the safety of a resident who is restrained in a chair in his room, how should the NA position the resident?
   (A) Close to the door
   (B) Differently every three hours
   (C) Next to a roommate
   (D) Near a call bell

7. What should the NA do to meet an alert resident's right for informed consent?
   - (A) Close the door and pull the curtain.
   - (B) Explain what is being done and why.
   - (C) Prevent a resident from leaving the facility.
   - (D) Get all consents in writing.

8. Which of the following is a right of a resident in a nursing home?
   - (A) Taking any medications they feel they need
   - (B) Refusing treatment ordered by the doctor
   - (C) Making as much noise as they want
   - (D) Demanding their meals at the times they prefer

9. Mrs. Glass is upset and goes into a long discussion about something that happened yesterday. What should the NA do?
   - (A) Listen for causes of the problem.
   - (B) Give an opinion about the problem.
   - (C) Tell her to tell you what is wrong.
   - (D) Interrupt and try to calm her down.

10. The NA helps a resident who has an above-the-knee amputation into a wheelchair. The resident starts to cry and says, "What good am I with this leg chopped off!" What should the NA say?
    - (A) "It wasn't chopped off, you had an operation."
    - (B) "You can still stand on your other leg."
    - (C) "It must be hard to adjust to losing a leg."
    - (D) "You'll get better when you get a new wheelchair."

11. Mrs. Brown had a stroke and is not able to move her left arm and leg. When the NA is dressing her, Mrs. Brown starts to cry and says, "I am useless since the stroke." What should the NA say?
    - (A) "It must be difficult not being able to move your arm and leg."
    - (B) "Cheer up. You will be able to move after physical therapy."
    - (C) "All people who have had a stroke feel this way."
    - (D) "Things will be OK after you feel better."

12. An NA will be getting married in two weeks. To involve the resident in the excitement of a wedding, what is the *best* thing the NA could say?
    - (A) "I know you can't go, but I'll bring you pictures."
    - (B) "Let me tell you all about my wedding plans."
    - (C) "Mrs. Shoemaker, tell me all about your wedding."
    - (D) "I am so excited, I can hardly wait for the big day."

13. A resident who was incontinent of urine says to the NA, "How can you stand this? It is such a messy job." What is the best thing the NA could say?

    (A) "I am used to it by now."
    (B) "It's not as bad as a bowel movement."
    (C) "This must be hard for you."
    (D) "It is part of my job."

14. The NA notes that a resident who usually talks a lot is being very quiet. What should the NA say?

    (A) "How come you are so quiet today?"
    (B) "You must be upset about something."
    (C) "What is wrong with you?"
    (D) "You seem very quiet today."

15. All of the following should be used to stimulate a totally blind resident EXCEPT:

    (A) A radio.
    (B) Flowers.
    (C) Animals.
    (D) Magazines.

16. Which of the following would be least stimulating to the deaf resident?

    (A) Magazines
    (B) A radio
    (C) Perfume
    (D) Holding hands

17. Which of the following is a true statement about communication?

    (A) A memo is a form of nonverbal communication.
    (B) A deaf resident cannot communicate with staff members.
    (C) Touch means different things to different people.
    (D) Words have the same meaning for all people.

18. What is one factor that is common to all communication?

    (A) It occurs in one direction.
    (B) There is transfer of a message.
    (C) Words are being used.
    (D) The people feel comfortable.

19. Which of the following is an example of nonverbal communication?

    (A) A birthday card
    (B) The use of touch
    (C) A telephone message
    (D) Noise in the room

20. When people are incontinent of urine or stool, what is it that makes them most upset?

    (A) The smell of the urine or stool
    (B) The feeling of being like a child
    (C) The fact that their skin gets wet
    (D) The feeling of being dependent

21. Psychosocial development is *most* affected by:

    (A) Diet.
    (B) Sleep.
    (C) Culture.
    (D) Oxygen.

22. How can the NA help meet a resident's need for self-esteem?

    (A) Comb and style the resident's hair.
    (B) Develop a close relationship with the resident.
    (C) Encourage the family to visit the resident.
    (D) Close the resident's window on a cold day.

23. Which basic human need is being met when the NA helps to reduce a resident's pain or discomfort?

    (A) Self-esteem needs
    (B) Safety and security needs
    (C) Physical needs
    (D) Love and belonging needs

24. The daughter of a dying resident says to the NA, "My mother was quite religious and was active in her church. She has a lot of faith." The NA's best response would be:

    (A) "Would you like us to pray for her?"
    (B) "Do you want us to call a minister?"
    (C) "Are you proud of your mother?"
    (D) "Do you have as much faith as your mother?"

25. After a month in a nursing home a Jewish resident says she misses lighting her candles on Friday night (Shabbas licht). The NA's best response would be:

    (A) "I'll ask the nurse if we can arrange that for you."
    (B) "Candles do have a peaceful effect."
    (C) "Habits are hard to break."
    (D) "The fire department will not allow it."

26. An elderly resident starts to cry and says, "My career came first and I hurt so many people along the way." The NA should understand that the resident most likely feels:

(A) Angry.
(B) Guilty.
(C) Hurt.
(D) Hostile.

27. A resident who has terminal cancer says to the NA, "I've been fairly religious, but sometimes I wonder if the things I did were acceptable to God." The NA's best response would be:

(A) "We all do both good and bad things in life."
(B) "If you are religious, you know God is forgiving."
(C) "You are worried about how God will judge you?"
(D) "Do you think you did as well as you could have?"

28. A resident who is dying says to the NA, "All my life I tried to be good and went to church, but I am still afraid of what happens after death." The NA's best response would be:

(A) "If you were good, you have nothing to fear."
(B) "Not knowing what the future brings can be scary."
(C) "God will appreciate that you went to church."
(D) "In life, all we have to do is try to be good."

29. A Catholic resident tells the NA that before getting ill she used to go to Mass and receive Communion every morning. The NA should ask the nurse to:

(A) Have the priest come and give her last rites.
(B) Assign her to a room with another Catholic resident.
(C) Arrange for her to receive Communion daily.
(D) Tell the resident the name of the nearest Catholic church.

Reasons for the answers

The asterisk (*) is in front of the correct answer.

1. *(A) This fails to support the resident's right to privacy and confidentiality; discussions must be among members of the health team directly responsible for the resident's care.
   (B) This action provides privacy and recognizes the resident's right to be treated in a dignified way.
   (C) Same as (B).
   (D) Same as (B).

2. *(A) This reduces fears and promotes safety; residents must know how to signal for help.
   (B) Important, but safety comes first.
   (C) Same as (B).
   (D) Same as (B).

3. (A) The resident should first know why he/she is being placed in a certain position.
   (B) This could be frightening if the resident does not know why it is being done.
   (C) The resident should first know why this is being done; this could be unsafe when the NA leaves to collect equipment.
   *(D) Residents have a right to know what, how, and why something is being done.

4. (A) This is a member of the health team who should know this information.
   (B) Same as (A).
   *(C) This would be against the resident's right to privacy.
   (D) Same as (A).

5. *(A) This supports confidentiality; resident information can only be shared with health team members.
   (B) This is done out of curiosity, which fails to support confidentiality.
   (C) The fact that a resident wears a wig is a private matter and should be kept confidential.
   (D) Joking about something that cannot be helped is embarrassing and demeaning to the resident and does not support confidentiality.

6. (A) Unsafe; no method has been provided for the resident to call for help.
   (B) This should be done every two hours, not three hours; this does not focus on the right to call for help.
   (C) While this may support social friendships, it does not provide for safety as roommates are not responsible for one another.
   *(D) Restrained residents should have a method for calling for help in the absence of a staff member.

7. (A) These actions support privacy, not informed consent.
    *(B) Informed consent means the resident knows what and why something is going to be done as well as who is going to do it.
    (C) This violates informed consent; an alert resident has the right to leave a facility.
    (D) Consents may be written or verbal; a verbal consent can be a gesture such as shaking the head yes or lifting up to get on a bedpan; legal written consents are obtained by the nurse.

8. (A) If done safely, self-administration of medications is allowed; however, medications must be ordered by the doctor.
    *(B) The resident has a right to refuse treatment; the doctor must inform the resident of the risks involved with no treatment.
    (C) Residents do not have a right to disturb the quality of life of other residents.
    (D) This is not practical; meals are usually scheduled during traditional mealtimes.

9. *(A) Listening is necessary for obtaining more information.
    (B) The NA should never give an opinion about a personal matter; the NA needs more information.
    (C) This cuts the resident off; the resident needs to explore her feelings; she may be anxious but not know why.
    (D) She will not calm down until she can talk about what happened.

10. (A) This challenges the resident, avoids feelings, and shuts off communication.
    (B) Same as (A).
    *(C) This identifies feelings and gives the resident a chance to talk.
    (D) This is false reassurance.

11. *(A) This focuses on feelings and gives the resident a chance to talk.
    (B) This denies feelings; false reassurance.
    (C) This is not true.
    (D) Same as (B).

12. (A) This reinforces the resident's sense of dependence and disappointment.
    (B) This is social chitchat; it does not focus on the resident.
    *(C) This allows the resident to relive a past event that was important in her life; it reinforces identity and self-esteem.
    (D) Same as (B).

13. (A) This response agrees with the resident's belief that it is a messy job, which may increase embarrassment; it does not focus on feelings.
    (B) Same as (A).
    *(C) This recognizes the resident's feelings.
    (D) Same as (A).

14. (A) This puts the resident on the spot and may cause a defensive response.
    (B) This is a conclusion that may be incorrect.
    (C) Same as (A).
    *(D) This statement identifies behavior and gives the resident the chance to talk, if desired.

15. (A) This stimulates the sense of hearing.
    (B) This stimulates the sense of smell.
    (C) This stimulates the sense of touch.
    *(D) The totally blind resident cannot see to read books or magazines.

16. (A) This stimulates vision.
    *(B) The deaf person cannot hear the radio, although vibrations may be felt.
    (C) This stimulates the sense of smell.
    (D) This stimulates the sense of touch.

17. (A) A memo communicates words in written form.
    (B) A deaf resident cannot hear but can still communicate through speech, gestures, sign language, the written word, etc.
    *(C) Touch does mean different things to different people, and how it is interpreted depends on age, sex, culture, the situation, and past experience.
    (D) This is not true; people place different values on words.

18. (A) Communication is an exchange between two people and is usually a two-way process.
    *(B) The purpose of all communication is to transfer meaning from one person to another.
    (C) Communication can be nonverbal.
    (D) In helping relationships, sad topics such as death and dying may make people feel uncomfortable.

19. (A) This is verbal communication; words are written.
    *(B) Nonverbal communication does not use words; touch, gestures, body posture, and facial expression are examples of nonverbal communication.
    (C) This is verbal communication; words are spoken.
    (D) This is sound that may or may not convey meaning; sounds that convey meaning are considered verbal communication.

20. (A) Although they may be embarrassed by the odor, it is the loss of control and feeling like a child that is most upsetting.
    *(B) Not being in control of urine or stool is a sign of returning to childlike behavior, which is upsetting.
    (C) Although being wet is uncomfortable, it is the loss of control and feeling childlike that is most upsetting.
    (D) Not all people who are incontinent are dependent; many are able to clean themselves.

21. (A) This affects physical needs, not psychosocial needs; diet is only one aspect of culture.
    (B) This affects physical needs, not psychosocial needs.
    *(C) Culture affects the way a person behaves and thinks about things and is considered psychosocial.
    (D) Same as (B).

22. *(A) This supports self-esteem because a nice appearance helps people to think well of themselves.
    (B) This supports the need for love and belonging.
    (C) Same as (B).
    (D) This supports a resident's safety, security, and comfort needs.

23. (A) This relates to the opinion one has of himself or herself.
    *(B) Preventing or relieving pain makes people feel safe; on Maslow's hierarchy of needs it comes after physical needs and before love and belonging needs.
    (C) Food, water, oxygen, elimination, and sleep and rest are basic needs that must be met first, to maintain life.
    (D) This relates to affection, closeness, and meaningful relationships with others.

24. (A) Not all members of the nursing staff might be willing to assume this role.
    *(B) This recognizes the content of the daughter's statement and may help to meet the resident's spiritual needs.
    (C) Not appropriate; this response is not related to the daughter's statement.
    (D) This is a probing question that could be viewed as a challenge.

25. *(A) The performance of religious rituals, if done safely, should be supported because they meet spiritual and emotional needs.
    (B) This does not recognize the religious importance of the candles and does not help the resident meet the need to perform this religious act.
    (C) This denies the resident's feelings and ignores the religious importance of lighting the candles.
    (D) Untrue; if performed safely, it can be done.

26. (A) Anger or hostility is expressed with blame and criticism.
    *(B) Sorrow and regret for past actions are related to feelings of guilt.
    (C) The resident was not hurt, but hurt others.
    (D) Same as (A).

27. (A) This does not focus on the resident's actual concern.
    (B) This denies the resident's feelings and may be false reassurance.
    *(C) This recognizes the content of the resident's concern; it restates what the resident said in a different way.
    (D) This puts doubt in the resident's mind and may increase anxiety.

28. (A) This denies the resident's feelings.
   *(B) This recognizes the resident's feelings.
    (C) This denies the resident's feelings and gives false reassurance.
    (D) Same as (C).

29. (A) This ignores the resident's need to go to Mass and receive Communion daily.
    (B) Unnecessary; the resident's spiritual needs must be met.
   *(C) Communion can be brought daily to the resident by a priest or lay minister of the Catholic Church.
    (D) The resident may not be able to follow through with this information; the nurse should communicate with the Church to have someone visit the resident.

ASSESSMENT OF THE RESIDENT

This section includes questions related to general physical assessment and specific questions about temperature, pulse, respirations, blood pressure, weight, and level of consciousness.

Questions

1. Name the vital signs.
   (A) Intake, output, and skin color
   (B) Level of consciousness
   (C) Temperature, pulse, and respirations
   (D) Height and weight

2. Which of the following should NOT be done when using an electronic thermometer?
   (A) Use the red probe for an oral temperature.
   (B) Take the thermometer into a resident's room.
   (C) Wash the hands before using the thermometer.
   (D) Use a new probe cover for each resident.

3. Of the following, when would a person's body temperature be at it lowest?
   (A) 6 AM
   (B) 11 AM
   (C) 4 PM
   (D) 8 PM

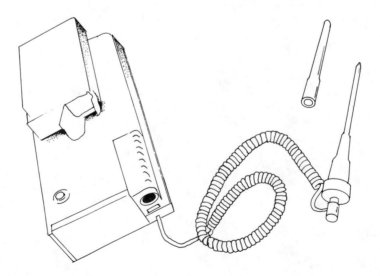

4. When taking a resident's vital signs, which vital sign can be taken with the piece of equipment shown on p. 136?
    (A) Pulse rate
    (B) Body temperature
    (C) Respiratory rate
    (D) Blood pressure

5. What is a normal rectal temperature?
    (A) 95.0° F
    (B) 97.6° F
    (C) 99.6° F
    (D) 101° F

6. When a resident drinks iced tea, how long should the nurse aide (NA) wait to take an oral temperature?
    (A) 2 minutes
    (B) 5 minutes
    (C) 15 minutes
    (D) 30 minutes

7. When taking a rectal temperature with a glass thermometer, which of the following should NEVER be done by the NA?
    (A) Turn the resident on the side first.
    (B) Let go of the thermometer when it is in the resident.
    (C) Shake down the thermometer before using it.
    (D) Report an abnormal temperature to the charge nurse.

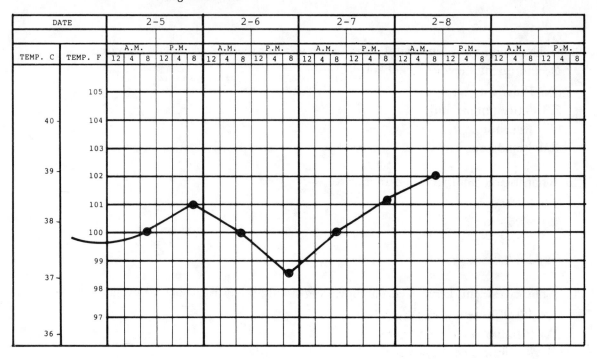

DATE		2-5		2-6		2-7		2-8			

8. On this graphic sheet vital signs are recorded every twelve hours. What was the temperature at 8 PM on February 7th?

(A) 98.6° F

(B) 100° F

(C) 101.2° F

(D) 102° F

9. A radial pulse rate measures the function of the:

(A) Arteries.

(B) Veins.

(C) Blood.

(D) Heart.

10. Which of the following vital signs should be reported to the nurse?

(A) Pulse rate of 72, oral temperature of 98.2° F

(B) Pulse rate of 82, respirations of 18 per minute

(C) Pulse rate of 92, oral temperature of 98.8° F

(D) Pulse rate of 100, respirations of 28 per minute

11. Which of the following vital signs should be immediately reported to the nurse?

(A) A pulse rate that is 80 and regular

(B) A respiratory rate of 36 per minute

(C) A rectal temperature of 99.6° F

(D) A blood pressure reading of 120/80

12. Besides a sphygmomanometer, what piece of equipment would the nurse aide need to take a person's blood pressure?

(A) Thermometer
(B) Glucometer
(C) Watch
(D) Stethoscope

13. Which blood pressure is normal in the elderly?

(A) 90/60 mm Hg
(B) 130/84 mm Hg
(C) 150/96 mm Hg
(D) 200/110 mm Hg

14. It is important to know a newly admitted resident's height to determine the:

(A) Need for an extra length bed.
(B) Resident's ideal body weight.
(C) Resident's clothing size.
(D) Height at which to set a walker.

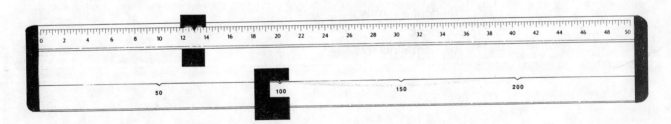

15. Mrs. Rogers is being weighed on a hospital-type scale. Using the drawing above, what should the NA record?

(A) 100 pounds
(B) 112.5 pounds
(C) 113 pounds
(D) 163 pounds

16. To get a correct weight with a standing scale the NA should do all of the following EXCEPT:

(A) Balance the scale before taking the weight.
(B) Write the weight down as soon as it is taken.
(C) Tell the resident to stand in the middle of the scale.
(D) Subtract the weight of the clothes from the weight.

17. The NA checks on Mrs. Green and finds her in bed with her eyes closed. Which of the following conclusions should be made by the NA?
    (A) The resident is sleeping.
    (B) Mrs. Green is unconscious.
    (C) More information is needed.
    (D) She is feeling withdrawn.

18. The best way to find out how Mrs. Palmer slept is to:
    (A) Ask the night nurse during report.
    (B) Ask Mrs. Palmer how she slept.
    (C) See if Mrs. Palmer looks tired.
    (D) Check the chart for this information.

19. An example of objective data is:
    (A) Pain.
    (B) Nausea.
    (C) Temperature.
    (D) Sadness.

20. The best source of information about a newly admitted alert resident is the:
    (A) Nurse.
    (B) Resident's family.
    (C) Resident.
    (D) Resident's doctor.

Reasons for the answers

The asterisk (*) is in front of the correct answer.

1. (A) These are not vital signs; intake and output measure fluid balance, and the skin reflects respiratory and circulatory functioning.
    (B) Although this reflects functioning of the central nervous system, it is not called a vital sign.
    *(C) Temperature, pulse, and respirations (TPR) are vital signs because they measure three basic functions of the body: body temperature, heart function, and breathing.
    (D) Height and weight reflect growth, nutrition, and fluid balance.

2. *(A) The red probe is used for rectal temperatures, and the blue probe is used for oral temperatures.
    (B) This is permitted as long as the resident is not on isolation.
    (C) This should be done to prevent the spread of microorganisms.
    (D) This should be done to limit the spread of microorganisms; a probe cover is immediately thrown away after use.

3. *(A) Body temperature is lowest in the morning by as much as 1 to 2 degrees F; it rises and falls over 24 hours and repeats this pattern every day; this is called a circadian rhythm.
    (B) It is not at its lowest; body temperature starts to rise as the day progresses.
    (C) Body temperature begins to peak between 4 and 7 PM.
    (D) The temperature is beginning to fall from its peak.

4. (A) A watch is needed to assess the pulse.
    *(B) An electronic thermometer can be used for oral, rectal, and axillary temperatures.
    (C) Same as (A).
    (D) A sphygmomanometer and stethoscope are needed to get a blood pressure reading.

5. (A) This is too low to be a normal body temperature.
    (B) This is within normal limits for an axillary (under the arm) temperature.
    *(C) This is within normal limits for a rectal temperature; the normal rectal temperature is 98.6° to 100.6° F (37.0° to 38.1° C).
    (D) This would be a fever.

6. (A) This is too short a time for the mouth to recover from the cold drink; the reading would be too low.
    (B) Same as (A).
    *(C) It takes 15 minutes for the mouth to recover from the cold drink and return to the resident's body temperature.
    (D) Unnecessary; this is too long a time.

7. (A) This exposes the buttocks for safe placement of the thermometer in the rectum.
   *(B) This would be unsafe and could harm the resident.
   (C) Before a temperature is taken, the mercury should be at the lowest mark on the scale.
   (D) Abnormal results should be reported to the charge nurse.

8. (A) This was the temperature at 8 PM on February 6th, not 8 PM on the 7th.
   (B) This was the temperature at 8 AM on both February 6th and 7th.
   *(C) This is correct.
   (D) This was the temperature at 8 AM on February 8th.

9. (A) Although an artery is pressed (palpated) to obtain a pulse, it is the heart rate that is being assessed, not the artery.
   (B) Veins do not expand and recoil with each beat of the heart.
   (C) Laboratory tests must be done to measure the functioning of blood.
   *(D) Each time the left ventricle of the heart contracts, it pumps blood through the circulatory system; the arteries, including the radial artery, expand and then recoil as blood is being pumped; this action can be felt and counted.

10. (A) These are within the normal range for these vital signs.
    (B) Same as (A).
    (C) Same as (A).
    *(D) These are above the normal ranges for these vital signs; normal pulse ranges between 60 and 100 beats per minute; normal respirations range between 14 and 24 breaths per minute.

11. (A) This is within normal limits.
    *(B) This rate is abnormal and should be reported; the normal respiratory rate is between 14 and 24 breaths per minute.
    (C) Same as (A).
    (D) Same as (A).

12. (A) This is used to take body temperature.
    (B) This is used to measure blood glucose levels.
    (C) This is used to take pulse and respirations.
    *(D) This is needed to hear the systolic and diastolic sounds of a blood pressure reading.

13. (A) This would be low blood pressure (hypotension).
    *(B) The normal range for blood pressure in the elderly is a systolic between 100 and 150 and a diastolic between 60 and 90.
    (C) This would be high blood pressure (hypertension).
    (D) Same as (C).

14. (A) This can be determined without an actual measurement.
   *(B) Ideal body weight is determined based on a formula of height and weight; this determines the number of calories a person needs in the diet.
    (C) Clothing size is mainly determined by weight and the number of inches around the waist and chest.
    (D) This is determined by the length of the legs and arms, not overall height.

15. (A) This is 13 pounds too low.
    (B) This is 0.5 pound too low.
   *(C) This is the correct weight; the large weight equals 100 pounds and the small weight is at 13 pounds.
    (D) This is 50 pounds too high.

16. (A) For a weight to be correct the scale must be balanced.
    (B) This prevents forgetting the weight.
    (C) This is necessary to keep the scale in balance.
   *(D) Residents should be weighed with the same amount of clothes each time.

17. (A) The NA does not have enough information to come to this conclusion.
    (B) Same as (A).
   *(C) To make a more valid assessment the NA must collect more information.
    (D) Same as (A).

18. (A) The nurse may not be totally aware of how well the resident slept.
   *(B) Unless confused, the resident is the primary and most reliable source of information.
    (C) This is inaccurate.
    (D) The nurse, who charts this information, may not have been totally aware of how well the resident slept.

19. (A) This is subjective because the resident must describe a feeling or sensation; subjective data cannot be measured objectively.
    (B) Same as (A).
   *(C) Temperature is measurable and therefore objective.
    (D) Same as (A).

20. (A) This is a secondary source.
    (B) Same as (A).
   *(C) The resident is the center of the health team and is a primary or major source of information.
    (D) Same as (A).

HEALTH AND SAFETY NEEDS

This section includes questions related to providing for the resident's general comfort, health, and safety, especially accident prevention, the use of restraints, infection control, and fire safety.

Questions

1. What is the most often used method for preventing a resident from falling out of bed?
   (A) Wrist restraints
   (B) Bedside rails
   (C) Sedative medications
   (D) Frequent checking

2. What is the main reason for accidents occurring in nursing homes?
   (A) Residents do not recognize hazards.
   (B) Residents sneak cigarettes.
   (C) Equipment breaks without warning.
   (D) Employees do not know safety rules.

3. The best way to keep a resident safe and prevent him from falling out of bed is by:
   (A) Telling him to call when he needs help.
   (B) Putting the bed in the lowest position.
   (C) Raising both side rails of the bed.
   (D) Placing an overbed table in front of him.

4. Which of the following actions is an example of poor body mechanics?
   (A) Leaning over from the waist
   (B) Bending the knees to pick something up
   (C) Holding an object close to the body
   (D) Spreading the feet wide apart

5. To avoid falls, the nurse aide (NA) should carry out all of the following actions EXCEPT:
   (A) Locking the wheels on equipment that moves.
   (B) Reporting loose floor tiles to the nurse.
   (C) Placing desired articles in easy reach of the resident.
   (D) Keeping residents in Geri-chairs.

6. When transporting a resident in a wheelchair, all of the following should be done to protect the resident *except*:
   (A) Maintaining the resident's hips back in the chair.
   (B) Keeping the resident's feet on the footrests.
   (C) Having the resident keep the hands on the arms of the chair.
   (D) Moving the resident's wheelchair onto the elevator with the small wheels first.

7. An occupied bed must be made for residents who:

    (A) Walk without help.

    (B) Use a wheelchair.

    (C) Sit in a Geri-chair.

    (D) Are on bed rest.

8. Why are restraints used?

    (A) To save the staff time checking on residents

    (B) To keep residents from wandering around the hall

    (C) To protect residents from hurting themselves

    (D) To reduce residents' agitated behavior

9. A restraint should be tied to the:

    (A) Side rail.

    (B) Headboard.

    (C) Bedside table.

    (D) Bed frame.

10. A doctor has ordered a vest restraint. To apply a vest restraint safely, what should the NA NEVER do?

    (A) Place the resident in a normal position.

    (B) Have the vest cross behind the back.

    (C) Tie the straps to the bed frame.

    (D) Secure the straps with a slipknot.

11. After applying restraints the resident gets agitated and more confused. What should the NA do?

    (A) Tell the resident to calm down and relax.

    (B) Remove the restraint until the resident calms down.

    (C) Isolate the resident in a quiet area.

    (D) Explain to the resident why the restraint is needed.

12. Confused, restrained residents may try to untie the restraints because they:

    (A) Are confused about what is happening.

    (B) Want to be in control of themselves.

    (C) Are attempting to keep the staff in the room.

    (D) May find the restraint painful.

13. When applying wrist restraints the NA should do all of the following EXCEPT:

    (A) Use a double knot to secure the straps.

    (B) Pad the wrists with something soft.

    (C) Tie the straps to the bed frame.

    (D) Place a call bell within reach.

14. Before doing any resident procedure, what should the NA do FIRST?
    (A) Clean the overbed table.
    (B) Pull the curtain closed.
    (C) Wash the hands.
    (D) Drape the resident.

15. The main reason the NA washes the hands before and after helping residents with bedpans and urinals and after emptying urinary collection bags is to:
    (A) Prevent the spread of microorganisms.
    (B) Be able to reuse equipment.
    (C) Promote emotional comfort.
    (D) Limit unpleasant odors.

16. What should NAs do to protect themselves from infection when assisting residents with perineal care?
    (A) Wash the hands before beginning.
    (B) Let the resident help himself/herself.
    (C) Wear clean gloves for perineal care.
    (D) Pour soiled water in the toilet.

17. Which of the following is most effective in preventing the spread of infection in a nursing home?
    (A) Isolation
    (B) Antibiotics
    (C) Sterilization
    (D) Handwashing

18. After handwashing, the water faucet should be shut off by the NA with:
    (A) The dirty hand.
    (B) An elbow.
    (C) A dry paper towel.
    (D) The towel used to dry the hands.

19. What is the main purpose of handwashing?
    (A) To prevent the spread of microorganisms
    (B) To make the hands look clean
    (C) To have the NA feel protected
    (D) To meet the facility's policies and procedures

20. How should the NA remove dirty linen from an occupied bed?
    (A) Shake out the crumbs.
    (B) Roll it into itself.
    (C) Push it together and make a ball.
    (D) Fold it from top to bottom.

21. A comb and brush should be washed:
    (A) Every time they are used.
    (B) Once a day.
    (C) Whenever hair is washed.
    (D) Once a month.

22. The most effective way to prevent the spread of the common cold in a nursing home is by:
    (A) Giving antibiotics to roommates of sick residents.
    (B) Teaching ways to prevent the spread of microorganisms.
    (C) Using strict isolation when a cold is identified.
    (D) Keeping the residents' doors closed during the winter.

23. When combing and styling a resident's hair, what should the NA NOT do?
    (A) Use a roommate's brush.
    (B) Brush the hair from the roots toward the ends.
    (C) Consider the resident's wants.
    (D) Brush small sections at a time.

24. Bacteria is known to grow best in places that are:
    (A) Hot.
    (B) Warm.
    (C) Cool.
    (D) Cold.

25. Mrs. Vane is on isolation. What is the MOST effective way to limit the spread of microorganisms by dishes at mealtimes?
    (A) Rinse them with hot water before returning them.
    (B) Use disposable dishes when possible.
    (C) Wash the dishes in the dirty utility room.
    (D) Transfer food into the resident's own dishes.

26. To clean a glass thermometer after use, what should the NA do?
    (A) Rinse it with hot water.
    (B) Soak it in alcohol.
    (C) Wash it with soap and cool water.
    (D) Wipe it dry with a gauze 4 X 4.

27. The main reason residents should not be allowed to smoke in bed is because it can:
    (A) Cause fires.
    (B) Annoy roommates.
    (C) Cause lung cancer.
    (D) Set off alarms.

28. When using a fire extinguisher, where should the NA point the hose?
    (A) Across the middle of the flames
    (B) Up and down the flames
    (C) Along the top of the flames
    (D) At the base of the fire

29. When a fire is discovered, what should the NA do FIRST?
    (A) Pull the alarm quickly.
    (B) Close the fire doors on the unit.
    (C) Remove residents from the immediate area.
    (D) Get the nearest fire extinguisher.

30. A class A fire extinguisher can put out a fire in a:
    (A) Maintenance closet.
    (B) Kitchen stove.
    (C) Toaster.
    (D) Bed.

31. To limit the danger of accidents due to smoking, what should the NA do?
    (A) Insist that smoking be done in smoking areas.
    (B) Encourage residents not to smoke.
    (C) Keep each resident's cigarettes at the nurses station.
    (D) Arrange for people who smoke to share bedrooms.

32. To prevent a resident from getting burned while smoking, what should the NA do?
    (A) Allow residents just one cigarette every hour.
    (B) Supervise residents when they smoke.
    (C) Keep cigarettes away from residents.
    (D) Light cigarettes for all residents.

33. Which of the following linens is NOT needed to change a bed?
    (A) Pillowcase
    (B) Spread
    (C) Draw sheet
    (D) Towel

34. What is the most important goal of making a bed?
    (A) To make a good-looking bed
    (B) To tuck in all the edges
    (C) To make the resident comfortable
    (D) To follow facility policy

35. Which of the following is NOT a rule of bed making?

   (A) Hold soiled linen away from the body.
   (B) Keep the top linens tight.
   (C) Make the bottom sheets free of wrinkles.
   (D) Use good body mechanics.

36. When making an occupied bed, what should the NA always do?

   (A) Make the draw sheet loose.
   (B) Leave the top sheet loose at the feet.
   (C) Use a waterproof pad under the buttocks.
   (D) Put two blankets on the bed.

Reasons for the answers

The asterisk (*) is in front of the correct answer.

1. (A) Not all residents need to be restrained; if necessary, a vest restraint is better; wrist restraints promote immobility, leading to bedsores and contractures.
   *(B) Bedside rails are barriers that provide security and prevent falls.
   (C) Sedation should never be used as a restraining measure; giving drugs is the role of the nurse, not the NA.
   (D) While this is important, it will not prevent falls.

2. *(A) Residents are often confused, use poor judgment, are disoriented, or deny physical limitations, resulting in accidents.
   (B) With proper supervision this does not happen.
   (C) Equipment usually shows wear and tear before breaking and should be repaired before it breaks.
   (D) Not true; all employees receive ongoing staff education about accident prevention.

3. (A) This is not a barrier to prevent falls.
   (B) This would not prevent a fall, but it would limit injury because the distance from the bed to the floor would be less.
   *(C) Side rails locked in place provide a barrier that prevents falls.
   (D) Unsafe; an overbed table has wheels that would roll and not provide a stable barrier.

4. *(A) This causes strain to the back and arms and should be avoided.
   (B) This reduces muscle strain because it uses the large muscles of the legs to lift.
   (C) This reduces strain by keeping the weight closer to the center of gravity.
   (D) This provides a more stable base of support.

5. (A) This keeps equipment from moving, which prevents falls.
   (B) Hazards should be reported and fixed to prevent falls.
   (C) This prevents reaching, which can cause a person to fall.
   *(D) A Geri-chair is a restraint and requires a doctor's order; residents need to be assisted to prevent falls, not be confined to a chair.

6. (A) This safely keeps the center of gravity back in the chair.
   (B) This supports the legs and limits pressure under the thighs and behind the knees.
   (C) This protects the hands and arms.
   *(D) Incorrect; always turn the chair around and enter the elevator with the large wheels first.

7. (A) A linen change can be done when the resi[dent]
    (B) Same as (A).
    (C) Same as (A).
    *(D) Residents on bed rest are not allowed out of bed; when[ ]
        while a person is in bed, it is called making an occupi[ed]

8. (A) Restraints should never be used for staff convenience.
    (B) Wandering is not a danger in itself if the person is able to wal[k]
    *(C) Restraints are used as a last resort to protect residents from hu[rting]
        themselves or others.
    (D) Residents may become more agitated after restraints are applied.

9. (A) Unsafe; the resident could get hurt if the side rail had to be quickly lowered
        in an emergency.
    (B) This is not a stable base of support; the line of pull could hurt the resident.
    (C) This is not a stable base of support because it can move.
    *(D) This is a stable base of support for the straps.

10. (A) This prevents extra stress or tension on muscles or joints.
    *(B) Unsafe; the back of the vest is high and if placed on backward, it can slide
        up around the neck and cause choking.
    (C) This safely secures the knot out of reach of the resident and provides a
        firm base of support.
    (D) This allows for quick release in case of an emergency.

11. (A) This denies the resident's feelings and does not address the cause of the
        agitation.
    (B) This would be unsafe.
    (C) Isolating a resident for agitation is not acceptable.
    *(D) Repeated explanations reinforce the reason for the restraint.

12. *(A) Confused residents do not have the mental ability to understand the
        purpose of the restraint.
    (B) Usually confused residents are not aware of the issue of self-control.
    (C) The purpose of their actions is to get free of the restraints, not to keep
        staff in the room.
    (D) If correctly applied and frequently checked, a restraint should not be
        painful.

13. *(A) A slipknot should be used so it can be easily untied in an emergency.
    (B) This is done to provide for safety.
    (C) Same as (B).
    (D) Same as (B).

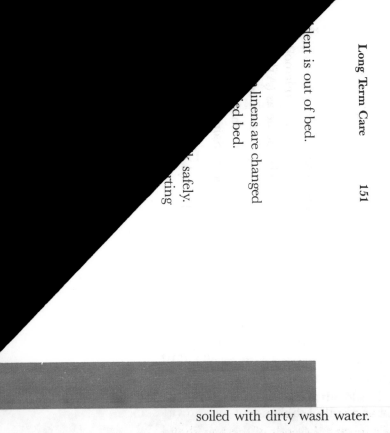

ached until the hands are washed to

thing in a room the NA should wash
ns.

taining the spread of microorganisms
ions.

own microorganisms; medical asepsis
ey do not spread to others.

emotional, needs.

ly after preventing infection.

microorganisms that might be on the

emselves; the NA may have to assist

A's skin and contaminated material;
rganisms.

protects the sink from becoming overly
soiled with dirty wash water.

17. (A) Isolation is effective once it is started; however, there may be disease-causing microorganisms present before the infection is diagnosed.

   (B) Usually antibiotics are not used to prevent infection, but to treat infection.

   (C) Sterilization is a process that destroys all microorganisms; however, only a small amount of equipment in a nursing home is sterilized.

   *(D) This is the single most effective measure that prevents the spread of microorganisms.

18. (A) Both hands are clean; the faucet is contaminated and a barrier is needed to shut it off.

   (B) This would contaminate the elbow.

   *(C) This provides a barrier between the clean hand and the dirty faucet, which prevents contamination of the hand.

   (D) The towel used to dry the hands is wet and does not provide an effective barrier; microorganisms can go through a wet paper towel.

19. *(A) Handwashing is the single most effective way to limit the spread of microorganisms from one person to another.

   (B) Hands can look clean but still be covered with disease-producing microorganisms.

   (C) Although handwashing does protect the NA, it primarily protects others from the NA.

   (D) This is an important policy and procedure; however, the hands are washed to limit the spread of microorganisms, not just to comply with a policy.

20. (A) Shaking linens spreads microorganisms into the air and should be avoided.
   *(B) This reduces loose ends and keeps soiled debris contained within the sheet.
   (C) This would have many loose ends and debris could fall on the floor.
   (D) This would be very difficult and uncomfortable for the resident who is in bed.

21. (A) Not necessary unless there is an unusual reason.
   (B) Same as (A).
   *(C) The hair should be washed weekly; to keep the newly washed hair clean, the comb and brush should also be washed.
   (D) Too long a time; this is not good aseptic practice because a comb or brush can harbor microorganisms and transfer them to newly washed hair.

22. (A) Antibiotics are usually given to treat infections, not prevent infections.
   *(B) Covering a cough or sneeze, washing the hands, and correct throwing away of used tissues can reduce the spread of microorganisms from one person to another.
   (C) Not necessary; this is only used for very contagious microorganisms.
   (D) This is not necessary; it isolates residents.

23. *(A) Never use a brush that belongs to another resident because it can spread microorganisms and cause hair and scalp problems.
   (B) This helps to spread normal oils toward the ends of the hair shafts.
   (C) This meets the resident's right for personal choice and supports a person's self-image.
   (D) This helps to remove knots and tangles while decreasing discomfort.

24. (A) Heat is used to destroy microorganisms (e.g., sterilization).
   *(B) Bacteria grows best in dark, moist, and warm places.
   (C) Microorganisms grow best in temperatures close to body temperature, 98.6° F.
   (D) Same as (C).

25. (A) Hot water is not enough to remove all microorganisms; the dishes would still be contaminated.
   *(B) Throwing away used paper or plastic dishes, knives, and forks uses medical asepsis to contain microorganisms.
   (C) The contaminated dishes cannot leave the isolation room without being double bagged.
   (D) Not practical; the dishes from the kitchen would still have to enter the isolation room.

26. (A) This would damage the thermometer's ability to take an accurate temperature.
   (B) This would cause an unpleasant taste in the mouth when used next.
   *(C) Soap and friction loosen dirt and microorganisms, while rinsing with cool water flushes the thermometer without causing it to break from excess heat.
   (D) This does not remove microorganisms from a used thermometer.

27. *(A) Residents who are confused, weak, or sleepy may drop burning ashes or cigarettes onto linens, which can cause a fire.
    (B) This is true, but it is not a fire safety problem.
    (C) Same as (B).
    (D) Just smoking in bed will not set off a fire alarm; alarms ring when a fire makes enough heat or smoke.

28. (A) This would scatter the burning material and spread the fire.
    (B) Same as (A).
    (C) The top of the flames is not the source of the fire.
    *(D) The base of the fire is where the fuel is burning; the source of the flames must be extinguished.

29. (A) This would be done after residents in immediate danger are removed.
    (B) This would be done after the fire alarm has been pulled.
    *(C) The first concern should always be the safety of residents in immediate danger.
    (D) Extinguishers can be brought to the scene of the fire after the residents are safe, the fire alarm is pulled, and doors to all rooms closed.

30. (A) A maintenance closet usually has flammable liquids; water would cause the chemical liquid to splatter, spreading the fire.
    (B) Water should not be used on a grease fire; water could cause grease to splatter, spreading the fire.
    (C) Water should not be used on an electrical fire because water conducts electricity.
    *(D) A class A fire extinguisher contains water and is used to put out wood, paper, or rag fires.

31. *(A) Smoking should be done with supervision in areas with adequate ventilation.
    (B) Residents have a right to smoke if done safely.
    (C) While this might be done with residents who use poor judgment, responsible residents should be permitted control of their own cigarettes.
    (D) Smoking is usually not permitted in resident bedrooms.

32. (A) This may not prevent burns; residents need to be supervised.
    *(B) Supervision of all smoking allows the NA to help residents when needed and prevent smoking-related burns.
    (C) Residents have a right to smoke as long as it is done safely and in a supervised smoking area.
    (D) Not necessary for all residents; residents who are able to light their own cigarettes safely should be allowed to do so with supervision.

33. (A) This is part of a complete linen change.
    (B) Same as (A).
    (C) Same as (A).
    *(D) Not necessary; a towel is needed for a bath, not a bed.

34. (A) A bed can look terrific but be wrinkled under the resident.
    (B) The sides and top of the top sheet and spread are not tucked in.
    *(C) This is always the first concern.
    (D) The resident's comfort comes first; hopefully, policies support resident needs.

35. (A) Good technique; this prevents transfer of microorganisms to uniforms and other surfaces.
    *(B) Top linens should only be tucked in at the feet and left to hang free at the sides; a toe pleat keeps the top linens loose over the feet.
    (C) Good technique; this reduces friction and skin breakdown.
    (D) This protects the resident and NA from injury due to straining.

36. (A) The draw sheet should be tight and wrinkle free to prevent a decubitus.
    *(B) This allows for movement and avoids pointing the toes, which could cause foot-drop.
    (C) This should only be used during a procedure such as perineal care or for a resident who is incontinent.
    (D) Not necessary; most facilities are maintained at a comfortable temperature, making two blankets unnecessary.

HYGIENE AND GROOMING NEEDS

This section includes questions related to personal care skills such as bathing, perineal care, mouth care, grooming, and dressing.

Questions

1. When giving a resident a tub bath the water should be:
   (A) 80° to 90° F.
   (B) 95° to 105° F.
   (C) 110° to 115° F.
   (D) 120° to 130° F.

2. If the nurse aide (NA) is assigned to do a partial bed bath, what should the NA do?
   (A) Ask the resident to wash as much as possible and then do the rest.
   (B) Help wash the resident's face, hands, underarms, back, and perineal area.
   (C) Ask the resident to wash the face, hands, and perineal area.
   (D) Help the resident to wash the whole body one part at a time.

3. Which of the following is true about bathing?
   (A) It reduces microorganisms on the skin.
   (B) Daily baths are needed for well-being.
   (C) Soap must be used for a bath to be effective.
   (D) Everyone likes to be clean and neat.

4. When bathing a resident, on what part of the body should the NA never use soap?
   (A) Eyes
   (B) Penis
   (C) Ears
   (D) Breasts

5. Which of the following is the correct temperature for bath water?
   (A) 90° F
   (B) 98° F
   (C) 110° F
   (D) 130° F

6. During a bath, the main reason the NA rinses after washing is to:
   (A) Improve circulation.
   (B) Remove soap.
   (C) Cool the resident.
   (D) Prevent pressure sores.

7. During a bed bath the NA can improve the resident's circulation by:

   (A) Using cool water for the bath.
   (B) Putting soap on the washcloth.
   (C) Using firm strokes toward the heart.
   (D) Keeping the window open during the bath.

8. A resident is incontinent of loose stools and is mentally impaired. What should the NA do to help prevent skin breakdown?

   (A) Frequently check the rectal area for soiling.
   (B) Wash the buttocks with strong soap and water.
   (C) Gently put a pad under the buttocks.
   (D) Place the call bell in easy reach.

9. When providing perineal care to a female resident the NA should do all of the following except:

   (A) Rub the area dry.
   (B) Wash from front to back.
   (C) Drape with linen.
   (D) Explain the procedure.

10. Which of the following is the best way to wash the female resident during perineal care?

   (A) In a circular motion
   (B) From front to back with each stroke
   (C) From side to side with each stroke
   (D) In an up and down motion

11. When washing the penis the NA should:

   (A) Rub the penis dry.
   (B) Use a lot of soap.
   (C) Wash under the foreskin.
   (D) Use hot water.

12. Women tend to get urinary infections more often than men because:

   (A) Women cannot use a urinal when voiding.
   (B) The urine flows toward the rectum when voiding.
   (C) Women use bedpans, which tend to grow bacteria.
   (D) The rectum is closer to the urinary opening.

13. An important action that supports a resident's dignity and self-image when giving denture care is:

   (A) Spreading a towel across the chest.
   (B) Closing the bedside curtain.
   (C) Using gauze to remove the dentures.
   (D) Lining the sink with paper towels.

14. The MOST important part of mouth care is:
  (A) Cleaning the tongue.
  (B) Using mouthwash.
  (C) Brushing the teeth.
  (D) Massaging the gums.

15. When providing mouth care for the unconscious resident the NA should:
  (A) Tell the resident to rinse with mouthwash.
  (B) Explain what will be done and why.
  (C) Use toothpaste and rinse with a lot of water.
  (D) Apply KY jelly (lubricant) to tongue and lips.

16. What is the most important action by the NA that will support healthy teeth?
  (A) Provide a balanced diet.
  (B) Brush teeth after eating.
  (C) Encourage a quart of milk a day.
  (D) Take the resident to the dentist.

17. When cutting fingernails, which of the following should be immediately reported to the nurse?
  (A) An injury caused by nail trimming
  (B) Dirt under the nails
  (C) Nail length after cutting
  (D) Calcium spots on the nail

18. Daily combing and brushing of hair prevents:
  (A) Head lice.
  (B) Tangles.
  (C) Oily hair.
  (D) Dandruff.

19. When styling a female resident's hair, what should the NA do FIRST?
  (A) Ask the resident how she would like it styled.
  (B) Start at the roots using long even strokes.
  (C) Use alcohol to remove tangled areas.
  (D) Part the hair down the back and make two pigtails.

20. People on complete bed rest tend to have which of the following problems with their hair?
  (A) Oily hair
  (B) Dry hair
  (C) Head lice
  (D) Matted hair

21. If a resident with diabetes complains about cold feet, what should the NA do?

    (A) Put snug socks on the feet.
    (B) Place a hot water bottle under the feet.
    (C) Wrap the feet in a blanket.
    (D) Use a heating pad around the feet.

22. To maintain safety when dressing and undressing a resident, which of the following should the NA do?

    (A) Take clothes off the weaker side first.
    (B) Bend joints within their normal range.
    (C) Put clothes on the stronger side first.
    (D) Offer the resident a choice of clothes.

23. A resident has a weakness on the right side. When planning to help the resident dress, what should the NA plan to do?

    (A) Encourage her to dress by herself.
    (B) Put her left sleeve on first.
    (C) Keep her in an open-backed gown.
    (D) Put her right sleeve on first.

24. Mrs. Jones is on a restorative grooming program. While assisting her with combing her hair the NA should:

    (A) Set time aside for a long teaching session.
    (B) Use a comb one time and then a brush the next time.
    (C) Offer constant support and encouragement.
    (D) Stop the session if she does not understand.

Reasons for the answers

The asterisk (*) is in front of the correct answer.

1. (A) This would be too cool, feel uncomfortable, cause chilling, and reduce circulation to the skin.
   (B) Same as (A).
   *(C) This is warm enough to feel comfortable and increase circulation to the skin.
   (D) This would be too hot and could cause damage to the skin.

2. (A) This would be a complete bed bath.
   *(B) These areas must be washed in a partial bed bath to control the growth of microorganisms.
   (C) Under the arms and the back must also be washed in a partial bed bath.
   (D) Same as (A).

3. *(A) Friction and use of water remove microorganisms and dirt from the skin.
   (B) Daily baths are not necessary; one bath a week plus daily perineal care and washing of the hands and face are enough under normal conditions; frequent baths can be very drying to the skin.
   (C) Soap is very drying and irritating to aging skin.
   (D) This is not a value held by everyone.

4. *(A) Soap can be irritating and injure the sensitive tissues of the eyes.
   (B) This area needs soap and water to remove urine and perspiration.
   (C) This area needs soap and water to remove earwax secretions.
   (D) This area needs soap and water to remove perspiration that collects on the skin under the breasts.

5. (A) This would be too cold and could cause a chill.
   (B) Same as (A).
   *(C) This is warm enough to increase blood flow, relax muscles, clean the skin, promote comfort, and not burn the skin.
   (D) This would be too hot and could hurt the tender skin of the elderly.

6. (A) Firm strokes improve circulation, not rinsing.
   *(B) Soap should be rinsed off the skin before drying because it is irritating and drying.
   (C) The resident should not be allowed to get a chill during a bath; a sponge bath to reduce a fever needs a doctor's order.
   (D) Relief of pressure is the most important measure to prevent pressure sores; keeping the skin clean and dry can help in preventing pressure sores as long as pressure is relieved first.

7. (A) This constricts blood vessels, which reduces circulation.
   (B) Not related to circulation; it removes dirt and sweat (perspiration).
   *(C) Firm strokes apply pressure on tissues, which helps return blood to the heart when stroked in the direction of the heart.
   (D) Same as (A).

8. *(A) Loose stool contains digestive fluids that are irritating to the skin and should be cleaned from the skin as soon as possible after soiling.
   (B) Strong soap can further irritate the skin.
   (C) This would not keep stool off the skin.
   (D) The resident is mentally impaired and is unaware of needs.

9. *(A) Rubbing can damage perineal tissue; the area should be patted dry with a towel.
   (B) This action moves dirt and microorganisms away from the urinary meatus and vagina toward the rectum; washing from clean to dirty is a basic principle of asepsis.
   (C) This helps to meet a resident's right to privacy.
   (D) When residents understand what and why something is done, they are less anxious and more able to help.

10. (A) This moves soiled material toward the cleaner areas of the vagina and urinary meatus.
   *(B) This action moves from the cleanest area (pubis) to the dirty area (rectum) and moves soiled material away from the urinary meatus and vagina.
   (C) Same as (A).
   (D) Same as (A).

11. (A) Rubbing should be avoided because it can cause an erection and embarrass the resident.
   (B) Soap is very irritating and drying to mucous tissue.
   *(C) Microorganisms and secretions collect under the foreskin, and these must be removed.
   (D) Warm water should be used because hot water can injure perineal tissues.

12. (A) Use of a urinal is unrelated to urinary tract infections; there are female urinals.
   (B) Stool being brought toward the urinary opening causes urinary infections, not urine flowing toward the rectum.
   (C) Women use the bathroom unless on bed rest; bedpans are cleaned to prevent the growth of microorganisms.
   *(D) Most urinary infections are caused by *Escherichia coli*, a microorganism found in stool.

13. (A) This protects clothes from soiling; it does not support dignity.
   *(B) This provides for privacy and supports self-image and dignity.
   (C) This does not relate to dignity; it allows for a better grip on the teeth when removing the dentures.
   (D) This does not relate to dignity; it prevents the dentures from breaking if dropped in the sink.

14. (A) This does not clean the teeth; it limits mouth odor.
    (B) This is not as effective as brushing.
   *(C) Food gets caught between teeth and along the gums and must be removed by brushing to prevent tooth decay and gum disease.
    (D) This does not clean the teeth; it supports healthy gums.

15. (A) An unconscious resident is unable to speak, respond, or help with care.
   *(B) Unconscious residents may be able to hear; care should always be explained.
    (C) Only small amounts of water should be used because of the threat of breathing it into the lungs (aspiration); toothpaste should be avoided because the unconscious person is not able to rinse the mouth.
    (D) Lubricants should only be used on the lips and nares (openings of the nose).

16. (A) This is helpful, but brushing and flossing the teeth are the best actions to prevent decay of the teeth and diseases of the gums.
   *(B) This removes debris and food particles from the teeth that cause tooth decay and gum disease.
    (C) Same as (A).
    (D) This is helpful, but a dentist usually treats or limits problems once they occur; daily brushing is the best way to prevent problems.

17. *(A) All injuries must be reported, documented, and treated.
    (B) This does not have to be immediately reported; the dirt should be removed during nail care.
    (C) Not as important as reporting an injury.
    (D) Not necessary; this is not important.

18. (A) Grooming the hair will not prevent head lice; it is caused by contact with lice or their eggs (nits).
   *(B) Combing and brushing separates strands of hair and carries secretions and oil down the hair shaft, preventing tangles and knots.
    (C) Washing will prevent oily hair, not combing or brushing.
    (D) Combing or brushing alone will not prevent dandruff; total hair and scalp care (such as washing the hair, rubbing the scalp, etc.) will help limit dandruff.

19. *(A) This allows for choices and supports the person as an individual.
    (B) Brushing or combing should start at the ends and work toward the roots to limit knotting.
    (C) This is drying and should be avoided.
    (D) This would violate a person's rights if done without permission.

20. (A) Bed rest is not related to the amount of secretions around the hair root/shaft; oily hair usually is a clue that the hair needs to be washed more often.
  (B) Bed rest is not related to the amount of secretions around the hair root/shaft; usually, dry hair is a clue that the hair needs to be brushed to spread natural secretions down the hair shaft.
  (C) Head lice or their eggs are transferred from one person to another, not caused by bed rest.
  *(D) Constant rubbing of the head against the pillow when moving around in bed causes the hair to get tangled and matted.

21. (A) This can reduce circulation, which can lead to skin ulcers.
  (B) This can cause burns in residents who have decreased feeling in the feet.
  *(C) This traps body heat and is the safest way to warm the feet.
  (D) Same as (B).

22. (A) Incorrect; this can put unnecessary strain on the weaker side; clothes should be removed from the stronger side first because the stronger side has greater range of motion.
  *(B) Correct action; joints stretched beyond their normal range can cause injury.
  (C) Incorrect; this would then cause muscle strain when trying to put clothes on the weaker side.
  (D) This supports the resident's right to make choices, not support safety.

23. (A) This may be very frustrating and tiring.
  (B) This puts too much stress on weak muscles.
  (C) Residents should be dressed in street clothes during the day.
  *(D) This puts less stress on weak muscles; the stronger side can stretch more easily to dress.

24. (A) Not effective; the resident can get tired and lose concentration during long sessions.
  (B) Use the same tool all the time because consistency is important; a brush may be easier to grasp.
  *(C) This helps to keep the resident motivated.
  (D) Repeating simple instructions may be necessary when there is a lack of understanding.

BODY ALIGNMENT AND MOBILITY NEEDS

This section includes questions related to the maintenance or restoration of resident mobility and the prevention of complications such as decubiti and contractures.

Questions

1. Which of the following is most important to report to the nurse about a resident who was ambulated.
   - (A) How long it took
   - (B) When it took place
   - (C) What was the response
   - (D) Where it took place

2. Which of the following is the safest way to assist a blind resident to walk?
   - (A) Hold his elbow while walking.
   - (B) Have him hold your arm.
   - (C) Have him use a white cane.
   - (D) Stand slightly behind him.

3. The safest position when lifting a resident is with the:
   - (A) Feet wide apart and one placed forward.
   - (B) Ankles and knees straight.
   - (C) Feet together and the knees bent.
   - (D) Knees straight and the waist bent.

4. To move a resident safely from a bed to a wheelchair, what should the nurse aide (NA) do?
   - (A) Get two more NAs to help.
   - (B) Lock the wheels of the wheelchair.
   - (C) Cover the resident's legs with a lap robe.
   - (D) Pull the curtain around the bed.

5. A resident must be transferred from a bed to a chair. What is the main reason for sitting the resident on the side of the bed for a few minutes?
   - (A) It allows time for the resident to rest.
   - (B) It gives the NA time to assist with shoes.
   - (C) It permits the resident to recover from feeling dizzy.
   - (D) It gives the resident an opportunity to put on a robe.

6. Which of the following is LEAST helpful in safely moving a resident from a bed to a wheelchair?
   - (A) Keeping the wheels of the wheelchair locked
   - (B) Using another person to help with the transfer
   - (C) Placing the wheelchair six feet away from the bed
   - (D) Putting shoes on the feet of the resident

7. What is the most important thing the NA must do when moving a person from a bed to a wheelchair?

   (A) Provide for the safety of the resident.
   (B) Lock the wheels on the bed and wheelchair.
   (C) Report to the charge nurse after the transfer.
   (D) Get another NA to help with the transfer.

8. The safest way to transfer an overweight (obese) paralyzed resident to a chair is with a:

   (A) Couple of NAs.
   (B) Hoyer lift.
   (C) Transfer belt.
   (D) Pull sheet.

9. The NA is transferring a resident from a bed to a chair. When the resident moves to a sitting position, what should the NA say to the resident to assess her response to the change in position?

   (A) "That was very good."
   (B) "Hold onto my shoulders."
   (C) "How do you feel now?"
   (D) "Did you enjoy your breakfast?

10. A device used to transfer a resident from a chair to a bed is a:

    (A) Transfer belt.
    (B) Cane.
    (C) Walker.
    (D) Vest restraint.

11. A resident has a weakness on the left side. When transferring this resident from a chair to a bed the NA should:

    (A) Have the resident put equal weight on both legs.
    (B) Use a mechanical lift (Hoyer lift) for the transfer.
    (C) Place the chair on the right side of the resident.
    (D) Position the resident's feet close together.

12. A resident on bed rest is on a turning/positioning schedule/clock every two hours. When the NA signs a signature/initial to the turning schedule, it means the:

    (A) Resident was turned at that time.
    (B) Resident's skin looks better.
    (C) Resident got range of motion to all joints.
    (D) Resident was told to turn over.

13. When positioning a resident in a side-lying position, which of the following actions by the NA would make the resident most comfortable?
    (A) Providing a blanket
    (B) Placing a pillow under the upper leg
    (C) Removing the pillow under the head
    (D) Using a footboard

14. In which position would a person most likely develop a decubitus at the base of the spine (sacral decubitus ulcer)?
    (A) Lateral (side-lying)
    (B) Sims' (three-quarters side-lying)
    (C) Prone (on the abdomen)
    (D) High Fowler's (sitting up in bed)

15. The main reason the NA turns a resident every two hours is to:
    (A) Reduce pressure.
    (B) Observe the skin.
    (C) Provide activity.
    (D) Relax all muscles.

16. When a person sits in a chair for a long period of time, what is a serious complication that can develop?
    (A) Flexion contractures of the hips
    (B) Lack of feeling in the arms
    (C) Boredom from the lack of activity
    (D) Loss of urinary bladder control

17. An Eggcrate mattress is a device used to:
    (A) Raise the lower legs.
    (B) Hold top bed covers off the feet.
    (C) Support the body in a normal position.
    (D) Spread pressure over a larger area.

18. Flotation pads or gel cushions relieve pressure by:
    (A) Increasing heat to the area.
    (B) Allowing air to circulate.
    (C) Limiting moisture.
    (D) Spreading body weight.

19. Which of the following is used to prevent a decubitus ulcer (bedsore)?
    (A) Eggcrate mattress
    (B) Urinary tube
    (C) Incontinence diaper
    (D) Range of motion

20. A sheepskin helps prevent decubitus ulcers because it:
    (A) Totally removes pressure on the buttocks.
    (B) Reduces rubbing against the bottom sheet.
    (C) Keeps the skin warm and moist.
    (D) Absorbs urine from the incontinent resident.

21. A plastic or rubber draw sheet should never be:
    (A) Directly against the skin.
    (B) Covered with a draw sheet.
    (C) Tightly pulled and tucked in.
    (D) Under the bottom sheet.

22. People are at high risk for developing a decubitus ulcer if they CANNOT:
    (A) Move.
    (B) Void.
    (C) Speak.
    (D) Hear.

23. Residents are at high risk for getting decubitus ulcers if they have:
    (A) Angina.
    (B) A stroke (CVA).
    (C) High blood pressure (hypertension).
    (D) A bladder infection.

24. The resident with the highest chance of getting a bedsore (decubitus) is the person:
    (A) Walking around.
    (B) Allowed out of bed.
    (C) On bed rest.
    (D) Who uses a wheelchair.

25. To make a bed that will help prevent bedsores, the bottom sheet should be:
    (A) Pulled tight.
    (B) Loose at the toes.
    (C) Changed every day.
    (D) Made with squared corners.

26. A decubitus ulcer (bedsore) is caused by:
    (A) Heat.
    (B) Gravity.
    (C) Aging.
    (D) Pressure.

27. Residents are at highest risk for skin breakdown when they are:
    (A) Unable to move.
    (B) Short of breath.
    (C) Confused.
    (D) Depressed.

28. Mrs. Cater is incontinent of urine and is on bed rest. She is at a high risk for developing a:
    (A) Joint contracture.
    (B) Urinary tract infection.
    (C) Decubitus ulcer.
    (D) Respiratory infection.

29. Contractures are caused by:
    (A) Too much pressure on the skin.
    (B) Prolonged flexion of a body part.
    (C) Lying in bed too long.
    (D) The aging process.

30. When doing range of motion (ROM) exercises for residents the NA should NOT move joints:
    (A) Beyond the point of pain.
    (B) Of unconscious residents.
    (C) That are paralyzed.
    (D) That have arthritis.

31. The NA provides passive ROM exercises mainly to prevent loss of:
    (A) Strength.
    (B) Muscle size.
    (C) Joint movement.
    (D) Muscle tone.

32. What is the main reason for ROM exercises?
    (A) Keeps joints moving
    (B) Limits muscle tone
    (C) Prevents bedsores
    (D) Helps breathing

33. When doing ROM exercises, opening a fist is called:
    (A) Flexion.
    (B) Abduction.
    (C) Opposition.
    (D) Extension.

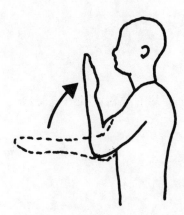

34. The NA is assisting a resident with ROM exercises. In the drawing above, what is the motion called?

    (A) Flexion
    (B) Hyperextension
    (C) Abduction
    (D) Rotation

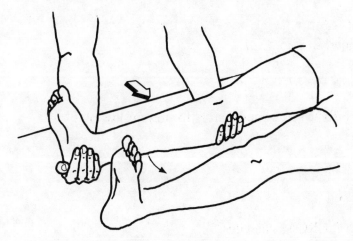

35. The NA is assisting a resident with ROM exercises. In the drawing above, what is the motion called?

    (A) Internal rotation
    (B) Flexion
    (C) Adduction
    (D) Pronation

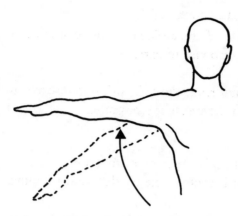

36. The NA is assisting a resident with ROM exercises. In the drawing above, what is the motion called?

    (A) Extension
    (B) Abduction
    (C) Supination
    (D) External rotation

Reasons for the answers

The asterisk (*) is in front of the correct answer.

1. (A) Although important, the response of the resident is more important because it assesses the resident's response to care.
   (B) Same as (A).
   *(C) This is most important because it addresses the resident's response to care given; future care will depend on the resident's response.
   (D) Same as (A).

2. (A) Unsafe; the resident should not lead because he cannot see.
   *(B) This allows the resident to follow; it protects the resident and promotes confidence.
   (C) This requires training and practice; many older people are unable to adjust to the use of a white cane.
   (D) Unsafe; this is used for residents who have impaired physical mobility, not for residents who are blind.

3. *(A) This provides a wide base of support for safety.
   (B) This places strain on the muscles of the back and should be avoided.
   (C) This provides a narrow base of support, which can result in a fall.
   (D) Same as (B).

4. (A) Not necessary; a Hoyer lift should be used if the resident is very dependent or heavy.
   *(B) This prevents the wheelchair from moving, which could cause an accident.
   (C) This provides for privacy and warmth, not safety.
   (D) This provides for privacy, not safety.

5. (A) This is not the main reason; it does not take a lot of energy to sit up.
   (B) Unsafe; this time should not be used to do any other activity because the resident may still be dizzy; shoes can be put on after it is determined that the resident is safe.
   *(C) When a person moves from a lying down to a sitting up position, blood drains from the head causing dizziness; time is need for the body to adjust.
   (D) Same as (B).

6. (A) This prevents the wheelchair from moving and is required during a transfer.
   (B) Two people provide more support than one and would be desirable.
   *(C) Unsafe; the resident might not be able to support the body weight for this distance.
   (D) Shoes support the feet and provide a firm surface for walking.

7. *(A) To be safe is a resident right; this includes the actions in the other answers.
   (B) This is only one part of a safe transfer.
   (C) This would be done after the transfer and would do nothing for resident safety.
   (D) Same as (B).

8. (A) Unsafe; the resident needs more support than two or three NAs can provide.
   *(B) This is the safest way to move an obese, dependent resident; the straps/hammock and the use of the lift provide the most support.
   (C) Unsafe; the resident needs more support than a transfer belt can provide; this is used for people who can support most of their weight.
   (D) This can help to move a resident up in bed or to turn, not to transfer.

9. (A) This does not get any information from the resident about how she feels since sitting up in bed.
   (B) This is a direction from the NA, not the collection of information from the resident.
   *(C) This is collecting information about the resident's response to care.
   (D) This is unrelated to the transfer.

10. *(A) This has handles for the NA to hold the resident safely during a transfer.
    (B) This is used for balance when walking, not during a transfer.
    (C) Same as (B).
    (D) A restraint is untied during a transfer; it is used to protect a person from falling out of a chair or bed.

11. (A) The weak leg cannot bear as much weight as the strong leg.
    (B) Not necessary; a resident with a weakness in one leg can assist with a transfer.
    *(C) This resident should get out of bed on the right side; the strong side can assist with the transfer.
    (D) Unsafe; spreading the feet apart widens the base of support and increases stability.

12. *(A) A signature/initial on a resident care flow sheet means that the assigned care was given.
    (B) This evaluation should be done by the nurse and recorded on the nursing progress notes.
    (C) A turning/positioning flow sheet documents when the resident's position was changed, not when range of motion was done.
    (D) Residents may be told or encouraged to turn but this does not mean it is carried out; the resident must be turned by the NA.

13. (A) This is only needed if the resident is cold.
    *(B) This increases comfort by supporting the weight of the upper leg and keeping the hips in normal alignment.
    (C) The head should be place on a pillow to keep it in normal alignment.
    (D) This is used when a resident lies on the back (supine position).

14. (A) No pressure is placed on the sacrum in this position.
    (B) Same as (A).
    (C) Same as (A).
    *(D) In the high Fowler's position most of the weight is placed on the buttocks and sacrum; weight causes pressure.

15. *(A) Skin can tolerate pressure for short periods of time without cell death from lack of circulation; turning reduces the pressure from body weight and permits blood flow to the area.
    (B) Although this would be done, the main reason a resident is turned is to relieve pressure.
    (C) Turning provides very little activity; active range of motion or other types of exercise provide activity.
    (D) Massage relaxes muscles, not positioning.

16. *(A) Sitting keeps the hips at a 90 degree angle, which promotes flexion contractures.
    (B) There should be free movement of the arms when sitting in a chair.
    (C) Sitting in a chair should not limit involvement with group or tabletop activities.
    (D) If toileted on request, a continent resident should not become incontinent because of sitting in a chair.

17. (A) Pillows are used to raise the lower legs, not an Eggcrate mattress.
    (B) This raises top covers off the feet and lower legs, preventing foot-drop.
    (C) Pillows or splints support the body in normal alignment.
    *(D) The Eggcrate mattress has raised areas that help to spread body weight more evenly over the body surface.

18. (A) These devices reduce friction and spread body weight; they do not have a heat source.
    (B) Air does not flow between the pads and the resident; they are filled with a gel-like material, not air.
    (C) These pads spread body weight, not limit moisture.
    *(D) Body weight is spread across the entire body part that is in contact with the pad/cushion, relieving pressure on the skin over the bony structures.

19. *(A) This reduces pressure by spreading the weight more evenly over the peaks in the mattress.
    (B) A Foley catheter should never be used just to promote clean skin and prevent a decubitus.
    (C) This will promote a decubitus because it keeps urine close to the skin.
    (D) This will prevent contractures, not a decubitus.

20. (A) Taking body weight off a part is the only thing that totally removes pressure.
    *(B) The soft tufts of lamb's wool reduce the friction that causes heat and damage to the skin.
    (C) Sheepskin keeps the skin dry by allowing air to pass between the tufts of lamb's wool; wet skin is likely to break down.
    (D) The purpose of sheepskin is not to absorb urine; it prevents friction and allows air to pass under the resident.

21. *(A) Plastic or rubber against the skin is hot and can cause sweating; moisture on the skin can cause skin damage.
    (B) This is a correct action to protect the skin.
    (C) This is a correct action; this prevents wrinkles, which would cause friction, pressure, and skin damage.
    (D) This still meets the need to have an absorbent, protective barrier between the rubber/plastic and the resident; however, it is more practical to place the rubber/plastic sheet between the draw sheet and bottom sheet.

22. *(A) Immobility causes prolonged pressure, which reduces circulation to body cells; the resident's position must be changed every two hours.
    (B) Not related to decubiti; people who cannot void may have overflow incontinence and may need a urinary drainage tube (Foley catheter).
    (C) The loss of this sense will not interfere with the ability to change position.
    (D) Same as (C).

23. (A) This is chest pain and does not cause pressure to the skin that could lead to a decubitus.
    *(B) This results in reduced mobility; when a person lies or sits in one position, the skin is exposed to pressure that causes bedsores.
    (C) This does not limit movement and therefore does not make a person more likely to develop a decubitus ulcer.
    (D) Same as (C).

24. (A) People who are out of bed have less pressure against the skin than those on bed rest.
    (B) Same as (A).
    *(C) Pressure causes a bedsore (decubitus), and people on bed rest tend to lie in one position.
    (D) Same as (A).

25. *(A) This gets rid of wrinkles that cause pressure and friction, which could result in a bedsore (decubitus).
    (B) The top sheet should be kept loose at the toes, not the bottom sheet.
    (C) If the sheets are clean and dry, they do not need to be changed daily.
    (D) Squared corners (mitered corners) are not related to bedsores because the sheets could still be wrinkled unless they are pulled tight.

26. (A) Heat causes burns, not decubitus ulcers.
    (B) Gravity is the physical principle that is related to accidents such as falls.
    (C) Skin changes related to aging may raise a person's risk of getting a decubitus, but they are not the cause of a decubitus.
    *(D) Pressure cuts off circulation and prevents oxygen from reaching the cells in the skin.

27. *(A) Paralyzed or unconscious residents can get bedsores from the weight of the body if allowed to be in one position too long.
    (B) Shortness of breath is not related to bedsores.
    (C) Confusion is not directly related to bedsores.
    (D) Depressed residents are still able to move around.

28. (A) Continuous flexion of a joint, not incontinence, causes contractures.
    (B) Microorganisms, not incontinence, cause urinary tract infections.
    *(C) Urine on the skin, which is irritating, and pressure related to bed rest can lead to skin breakdown.
    (D) Increased mucus that cannot be coughed up and microorganisms cause respiratory infections.

29. (A) This causes decubitus ulcers, not contractures.
    (B) Contractures will not develop if residents on bed rest do range of motion exercises and are positioned in normal body alignment.
    *(C) This permits shortening of the flexor muscles and lengthening of the extensor muscles, resulting in contractures.
    (D) Immobility, not aging, causes contractures.

30. *(A) Pain indicates that there is strain on the muscles or joints, and ROM of that joint should be stopped.
    (B) Unconscious people cannot move and are at high risk of developing contractures; ROM should be done.
    (C) The muscles are paralyzed, not the joints; these joints must receive ROM.
    (D) People with arthritis must do ROM several times a day to limit stiffness and prevent contractures.

31. (A) This is done by active exercise (isotonic exercise).
    (B) Same as (A).
    *(C) ROM flexes and extends muscles, which prevents contractures.
    (D) Same as (A).

32. *(A) Opening (extending) and bending (flexing) a joint prevents rigid joints (contractures).
    (B) ROM increases muscle tone.
    (C) ROM is not related to bedsores; reducing pressure prevents bedsores, not ROM.
    (D) Aerobic exercises or breathing exercises help breathing, not ROM.

33. (A) This would be making a fist.
    (B) This would be spreading the fingers apart.
    (C) This would be touching the thumb to the tip of each finger, not extension.
    *(D) Straightening out a joint is called extension.

34. *(A) Flexion occurs when the angle of the joint is made smaller by bending a body part.
    (B) This is excessive straightening of a joint, not flexion.
    (C) This is moving a body part away from the center of the body, not flexion.
    (D) This is rolling or turning a joint around an axis, not flexion.

35. (A) This is turning a joint inward, not adduction.
    (B) This is making the angle of a joint smaller by bending a body part.
    *(C) Correct; this is moving a body part toward the center of the body.
    (D) This is turning a body part downward, not adduction.

36. (A) This occurs when a body part is straightened, not abducted.
    *(B) Correct; this is moving a body part away from the center of the body.
    (C) This is turning a body part upward, not abduction.
    (D) This is turning the joint outward, not abduction.

NUTRITION AND FLUID BALANCE NEEDS

This section includes questions related to normal nutrition, problems that interfere with adequate nutrition, dietary instructions, tube feedings, fluid balance, and intake and output.

Questions

1. What is the main cause of obesity (overweight)?
   (A) An intake of more calories than are burned for energy
   (B) A serious mental condition causing overeating
   (C) A problem with glands preventing loss of weight
   (D) Diabetes, which prevents the breakdown of sugar

2. When the amount of calories eaten does not meet energy needs, a resident will:
   (A) Void (urinate) less.
   (B) Lose weight.
   (C) Have respiratory distress.
   (D) Become thirsty.

3. The doctor orders 1,000 cc (ml) fluid restriction a day for a resident. What should the nurse aide (NA) do?
   (A) Provide fluid based on the fluid restriction plan.
   (B) Give fluids just during mealtimes.
   (C) Encourage just clear fluids.
   (D) Put a sign at the bedside stating "restrict fluids."

4. Which of the following would have to be measured if the resident was on intake and output (I&O)?
   (A) Applesauce
   (B) Ice cream
   (C) Rice pudding
   (D) Pureed fruits

5. When a resident is on I&O, what should the NA do?
   (A) Measure the amount of fluid the resident drinks and urinates.
   (B) Keep the resident in a vest restraint most of the time.
   (C) Get the resident out of bed and to the day room every day.
   (D) Make sure the resident's diet is low in salt.

DAILY INTAKE AND OUTPUT RECORD

RESIDENT NAME: DATE:

11-7 FLUID INTAKE			11-7 FLUID OUTPUT			COMMENTS
TIME	AMOUNT	TYPE	TIME	AMOUNT	TYPE	
12:00	140	Juice				
1:00	120	water	1:00	320	urine	
5:00	300	coffee	3:00	200	urine	
7:00	300	water	5:00	100	urine	
			6:00	60	Vomitus	
TOTAL:			TOTAL:			

6. A resident is on I&O. According to the I&O record above, what would be the total output during the 11 to 7 shift?
   (A) 420 cc (ml)
   (B) 860 cc (ml)
   (C) 620 cc (ml)
   (D) 680 cc (ml)

7. What form is used to record how much water a person drinks?
   (A) Nurse's notes
   (B) NA assignment sheet
   (C) I&O record
   (D) Weight book

8. The doctor orders forced fluids. To increase a resident's intake of fluid, what should the NA do?
   (A) Make him drink four ounces of fluid every hour.
   (B) Offer him fluids he likes and encourage him to drink.
   (C) Explain that he must drink or a feeding tube will be used.
   (D) Measure and record on the I&O record everything he drinks.

9. NPO means a person:
   (A) Should just drink clear fluids.
   (B) Is on complete bed rest.
   (C) Can have nothing by mouth.
   (D) Has a low salt diet.

10. If a person on I&O drinks 12 ounces of milk, the NA should mark on the resident's record an intake of:
    (A) 30 cc (ml).
    (B) 90 cc (ml).
    (C) 240 cc (ml).
    (D) 360 cc (ml).

11. The NA must feed a helpless resident. What should the NA do to prevent the resident from choking?
    (A) Allow the resident time to empty the mouth after each spoonful.
    (B) Ask the resident to direct the order of food served.
    (C) Pace the meal so that the resident can talk with the NA.
    (D) Serve only pureed and soft foods to the resident.

12. A resident had a stroke (CVA) and has left-sided weakness. When feeding the resident the NA should do all of the following except:
    (A) Sit the resident in an upright position.
    (B) Tell the resident to think about swallowing.
    (C) Place soft food on the weak side of the mouth.
    (D) Put food toward the back of the mouth.

13. When feeding a resident who is short of breath, what should the NA do?
    (A) Allow for short rest periods.
    (B) Avoid using a straw.
    (C) Feed the resident quickly.
    (D) Tie a bib around the neck.

14. A resident has difficulty swallowing. To prevent choking after the feeding, what should the NA do?
    (A) Rinse the dentures.
    (B) Check the mouth for food.
    (C) Leave water at the bedside.
    (D) Keep the dessert for later.

15. When a resident throws up (vomits), what should the NA do with the material thrown up (vomitus)?
    (A) Flush it down the toilet.
    (B) Pour it down the sink.
    (C) Have the nurse look at it.
    (D) Throw it in the medical waste garbage can.

16. When a resident is vomiting in bed, in which of the following positions should the NA place the resident's head?
    (A) Over the toilet
    (B) To the side
    (C) Over the sink
    (D) Forward and between the knees

17. When a resident complains of nausea, what should the NA do to support comfort?

    (A) Hold all meals.
    (B) Give frequent mouth care.
    (C) Provide an emesis basin.
    (D) Force fluids.

18. A resident is on a special diet that has between-meals snacks (supplements). The NA should serve the snack when:

    (A) It is ordered to be given.
    (B) It arrives on the unit.
    (C) The resident asks for the snack.
    (D) There is time between meals.

19. A resident is overweight and is on a reduced calorie diet. The NA can help the resident lose weight by doing all of the following EXCEPT:

    (A) Praising the resident when weight is lost.
    (B) Encouraging low calorie snacks.
    (C) Telling the resident to avoid breakfast.
    (D) Teaching the resident to chew and eat slowly.

20. Mr. Marshall is holding a lot of fluid in his feet and ankles and is very overweight. What kind of diet should the NA expect the doctor to order?

    (A) Low salt, low calorie
    (B) Low salt, low protein
    (C) High salt, low calorie
    (D) High salt, low protein

21. The resident is on a low sodium diet. Which of the following should the NA teach the family not to bring for the resident?

    (A) Diet soda
    (B) Green apples
    (C) Uncooked carrots
    (D) Hard candy

22. The resident is on a low sodium diet. The lunch tray arrives. Which of the following items on the tray should the NA remove?

    (A) Sugar
    (B) Salt
    (C) Fluids
    (D) Butter

23. A tube that enters the nose for the purpose of feeding a resident goes into the:
    (A) Lungs.
    (B) Stomach.
    (C) Colon.
    (D) Trachea.

24. The NA must give personal care to a resident receiving a tube feeding. To prevent the feeding from entering the breathing passages (aspiration), what should the NA do?
    (A) Keep the head of the bed elevated when the feeding is running.
    (B) Shut off the tube feeding when giving personal care.
    (C) Provide frequent mouth care between tube feedings.
    (D) Keep the tube feeding bag lower than the head of the bed.

25. A resident has a nasogastric tube for tube feedings. When providing a bed bath, which of the following needs special care?
    (A) The feet
    (B) The mouth
    (C) The back
    (D) The hands

Reasons for the answers

The asterisk (*) is in front of the correct answer.

1. *(A) If more calories are taken in than the body needs for energy, it will be converted to fat, which causes weight gain.
   (B) You do not need to suffer from a serious mental condition to overeat.
   (C) A small percentage of people suffer from obesity due to problems with the glands.
   (D) Diabetes is a disease affecting sugar metabolism and is not the cause of obesity.

2. (A) This is related to not enough fluid intake or kidney disease.
   *(B) When body fat is used for energy, a person will lose weight.
   (C) Not directly related; if very anemic, a person could tire easily.
   (D) This is related to not enough fluid intake, not calorie intake.

3. *(A) The 1,000 cc (ml) of fluid intake should be divided over 24 hours in a formal plan that is followed.
   (B) A schedule for fluid intake should be spread over the waking hours, not just given with meals.
   (C) Fluid restriction relates to total amount of fluid taken in each day, not the type of fluid.
   (D) This violates the resident's right to privacy.

4. (A) This is a solid.
   *(B) Ice cream changes from a solid to a liquid when it melts.
   (C) Same as (A).
   (D) Same as (A).

5. *(A) I&O stands for intake and output; the amount of fluid the resident takes in and puts out is measured to compute fluid balance.
   (B) Unrelated to I&O.
   (C) Same as (B).
   (D) Same as (B).

6. (A) This is the total water intake.
   (B) This is the total fluid intake.
   (C) This is the total urinary output.
   *(D) The urinary output (620) plus the vomitus (60) equals a total output of 680 cc.

7. (A) The nurses record assessments and care given on this form.
   (B) This is used to direct care and in some cases document grooming and other care given by the NA.
   *(C) All fluid intake and fluid losses are measured and recorded on an I&O sheet.
   (D) A weight book is used to record a resident's weight, not the I&O of fluid.

8. (A) Making a person do something is the use of force and increases the feeling of helplessness; the resident should be taught and encouraged.

   *(B) The resident will most likely drink if he likes the fluid offered and is encouraged.

   (C) This is a threat and is unacceptable.

   (D) While this must be done, it is done after the resident drinks.

9. (A) This is a clear fluid diet, not NPO.

   (B) Complete bed rest could be written as CBR, not NPO.

   *(C) Non Per Os (NPO) means nothing by mouth.

   (D) A low sodium diet could be written as a low Na diet, not NPO.

10. (A) This is only 1 ounce and would be too little.

    (B) This is only 3 ounces and would be too little.

    (C) This is only 8 ounces and would be too little.

    *(D) One ounce is equal to 30 cc (ml); 12 times 30 equals 360 cc (ml).

11. *(A) This prevents food from building up in the mouth; it does not rush the resident.

    (B) This supports choices and control by the resident; it does not prevent choking.

    (C) Pacing the meal is done for rest periods, not to provide time for talking; talking with food in the mouth can cause choking.

    (D) The helpless resident may not have difficulty swallowing and may be allowed a regular diet.

12. (A) This uses gravity to move food down the esophagus and is desirable.

    (B) The resident's thinking about the task can help her do the task better.

    *(C) This can cause choking; muscle weakness prevents controlling the movement of food to the back of the mouth.

    (D) This requires less effort to swallow the food and is desirable.

13. *(A) This allows time to rest and breathe; the process of eating uses energy.

    (B) A straw can be helpful; it requires less energy than drinking from a cup.

    (C) This will cause more shortness of breath; activity increases the need for oxygen.

    (D) The resident is short of breath and is not a person who needs a bib.

14. (A) Although this should be done, it does not limit the threat of choking from debris trapped on the weak side of the mouth.

    *(B) Food can become trapped in the mouth because of muscle weakness; this could cause choking after the meal is finished.

    (C) Food or fluid should not be left at the bedside; residents who have difficulty swallowing should be supervised when drinking or eating.

    (D) The dessert should be part of the meal; this would not limit choking.

15. (A) Vomitus should be measured and then assessed by the nurse before it is flushed down the toilet.
    (B) The sink is not an acceptable place to discard vomitus; it should be measured, assessed by the nurse, and then flushed down the toilet.
    *(C) Color, odor, and consistency of vomitus can indicate specific problems; therefore, it should be assessed by the nurse.
    (D) Vomitus does not have to be disposed of with medical waste; it can be safely flushed down the toilet.

16. (A) This could cause a fall because it alters balance; vomiting takes energy and can make a person weak.
    *(B) This helps drain the mouth of vomitus and reduces the threat of choking.
    (C) Same as (A).
    (D) This position is sometimes used to increase blood to the brain when a person feels dizzy.

17. (A) This is not appropriate; nausea may last for days.
    (B) Regular daily mouth care is adequate; more frequent mouth care is done when a resident is vomiting.
    *(C) This provides emotional comfort; it reduces the fear of becoming soiled or soiling the linen.
    (D) Regular fluid intake is adequate.

18. *(A) Supplements/snacks should be served when ordered; they should not interfere with meals.
    (B) They may arrive on the unit long before they should be given.
    (C) Residents may have little appetite and may never ask for a snack; they should be given as ordered.
    (D) Between-meal supplements should be given on time, not just when there is time.

19. (A) This is encouraging and keeps the resident motivated.
    (B) This helps to keep caloric intake low.
    *(C) Residents should eat all the food on the tray when on a special diet; meals should not be skipped.
    (D) This makes a meal seem longer and allows the body to feel more full.

20. *(A) Salt holds water and increased calories add to body weight; therefore, both should be avoided.
    (B) Protein is not related to his problem.
    (C) High salt would increase fluid retention and should be avoided.
    (D) Same as (C).

21. *(A) Diet soda contains sodium.
    (B) Fresh fruit usually does not contain sodium.
    (C) These are low in sodium.
    (D) Same as (C).

22. (A) Not related to sodium; sugar would be avoided or controlled on a low calorie or American Diabetes Association (ADA) diet.
    *(B) Table salt contains sodium, which is not allowed on a low sodium diet.
    (C) Fluids that do not contain sodium are allowed; fluids should be avoided when a resident is on fluid restriction, not a low sodium diet.
    (D) This should be avoided when a resident is on a low fat diet, not a low sodium diet.

23. (A) The lungs are organs of respiration, not digestion.
    *(B) The tube goes into the nose, down the esophagus, and into the stomach.
    (C) This refers to the large intestines at the end of the digestive tract; first, food has to go through the stomach and small intestines.
    (D) This is the breathing passage that connects the mouth and nose to the bronchi that lead to the lungs; this is part of the respiratory system.

24. *(A) This allows fluid to enter and stay in the stomach through the principle of gravity.
    (B) Never shut off a tube feeding because this is the role of the nurse; when possible, provide care around the feeding schedule.
    (C) This keeps the mucous membranes of the mouth clean and moist; it does not prevent aspiration.
    (D) The tube feeding bag height is adjusted by the nurse, not the NA; the bag should be higher than the place it enters the body.

25. (A) The care given to this area during a normal bed bath would be enough.
    *(B) The mouth is dry because the person is not chewing food, which normally increases the amount of saliva.
    (C) Same as (A).
    (D) Same as (A).

BOWEL AND BLADDER ELIMINATION NEEDS

This section includes questions related to such topics as toileting, incontinence, constipation, diarrhea, enemas, bowel and bladder training, and care of residents with urinary catheters.

Questions

1. Mrs. Ambrosio asks to use the bedpan. The nurse aide (NA) should:
    (A) Tell the resident to try to hold it longer.
    (B) Place the resident on the bedpan in a sitting position.
    (C) Check the time to see if the resident can void.
    (D) Pour warm water over the perineal area.

2. A resident in a wheelchair asks to go to the bathroom even though she only voided one-half hour ago. What should the NA do?
    (A) Explain that she just went one-half hour ago.
    (B) Take her to her room and put her on a bedpan.
    (C) Encourage her to hold it for two more hours.
    (D) Take her to the bathroom and put her on the toilet.

3. Some residents cannot always control their urine. To help a resident be continent, what should the NA do?
    (A) Tell him to stay in his room.
    (B) Toilet him every two hours.
    (C) Limit his fluid intake.
    (D) Apply disposable diapers.

4. Why do elderly people most often become incontinent of urine?
    (A) The muscles related to urination become weak.
    (B) They do not drink enough fluids each day.
    (C) They want to control others by their actions.
    (D) Their diets do not have enough fiber.

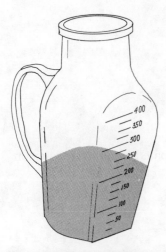

5. A resident on intake and output (I&O) urinates. According to the urinal pictured above, how many cubic centimeters (cc), or milliliters (ml), should the NA record on the I&O record?

(A) 175 cc (ml)
(B) 200 cc (ml)
(C) 250 cc (ml)
(D) 300 cc (ml)

6. A person who drinks large amounts of fluid will:

(A) Have dark-colored urine.
(B) Overwork the kidneys.
(C) Have to urinate more often.
(D) Stretch the bladder too much.

7. How would a person's urine look if the person drinks less than a normal amount of fluid?

(A) Dark yellow
(B) Cloudy
(C) Pink tinged
(D) Straw colored

8. When a person's urine output is less than the fluid intake, the person will:

(A) Gain weight.
(B) Become incontinent.
(C) Get diarrhea.
(D) Urinate more often.

9. Black, tarry-colored stools are related to:
  (A) Constipation.
  (B) Bleeding.
  (C) Diarrhea.
  (D) Gas.

10. A tap water enema is usually given to:
  (A) Empty the bowel of stool.
  (B) Drain the urinary bladder.
  (C) Limit nausea and vomiting.
  (D) Reduce abdominal gas.

11. The resident who would MOST likely become constipated would be the person who:
  (A) Drinks 3,000 cc (ml) of fluid a day.
  (B) Likes to sit and watch TV most of the day.
  (C) Eats bran cereal for breakfast every day.
  (D) Gets a pill to prevent constipation once a day.

12. Which of the following steps comes first in a bladder retraining program?
  (A) Offer the bedpan every two hours.
  (B) Provide fluids every two hours and with meals.
  (C) Find out the resident's usual voiding pattern.
  (D) Give the bedpan whenever the resident asks for it.

13. What is the first step in a bladder retraining program?
  (A) Find out the resident's usual voiding pattern.
  (B) Offer the resident the bedpan every two hours.
  (C) Make sure the resident can cooperate.
  (D) Give enough fluids to the resident.

14. When ambulating a resident with a urinary catheter, what should the NA do?
  (A) Hang the bag on an IV pole.
  (B) Hold the bag below the level of the bladder.
  (C) Use a clamp to stop the flow of urine.
  (D) Disconnect the tube from the bag.

15. A resident with a urinary tube (Foley catheter) is placed in a wheelchair. What should the NA do with the drainage bag?
  (A) Place it in the resident's lap.
  (B) Hang it from the handgrips of the wheelchair.
  (C) Put it on the floor under the wheelchair.
  (D) Hook it on the side of the chair below the bladder.

16. The resident has a urinary catheter (Foley), but the bed is always wet when the NA cares for the resident. What should the NA do?

    (A) Tell the nurse about the situation with the resident.
    (B) Wash and dry the resident when it happens.
    (C) Place a disposable underpad under the resident.
    (D) Ask the resident to call when she has the urge to void.

17. When changing a condom catheter (external catheter) the NA should do all of the following except:

    (A) Roll the condom up the shaft of the penis.
    (B) Moisten the penis before putting on the condom.
    (C) Keep the tubing from getting caught under the legs.
    (D) Hang the drainage bag on the bed frame.

Reasons for the answers

The asterisk (*) is in front of the correct answer.

1. (A) The resident may not be able to wait.
   *(B) The resident has a right to have needs met; sitting is the normal position for elimination by a female.
   (C) The resident has a right to have needs met regardless of the schedule.
   (D) Not necessary; the resident has stated that she needs to void.

2. (A) This denies the resident's need to urinate.
   (B) The resident should be assisted to the bathroom, which permits a more normal position for urination.
   (C) The resident has said she needs to urinate; this is too long a period of time to wait.
   *(D) This accepts the resident's need to urinate and promotes control; when possible, the toilet instead of a bedpan should be used because it is more comfortable and normal.

3. (A) This would promote isolation and should be avoided.
   *(B) A routine toileting program increases muscle control of the bladder and empties the bladder of urine.
   (C) This could result in bladder infections; fluids are needed for life and to keep the kidneys functioning.
   (D) This should be avoided; this would encourage incontinence and make the resident feel like a child.

4. *(A) Muscles tend to lose strength and flexibility as they age.
   (B) The amount of fluid intake is not related to incontinence.
   (C) This is untrue in relation to urination; most people want to be in control of their body functions.
   (D) Fiber is related to elimination of stool, not urinary elimination.

5. (A) Incorrect; this is too low.
   *(B) This is the correct measurement.
   (C) Incorrect; this is too high.
   (D) Same as (C).

6. (A) This would most often happen if a person had a small fluid intake.
   (B) The kidney's job is to maintain fluid balance; extra fluid intake would only be a stress for those people with kidney problems.
   (C) The kidneys maintain fluid balance; the more fluid the person drinks, the more the person will urinate.
   *(D) The person would have the urge to urinate before the bladder becomes overstretched.

7. *(A) With a small fluid intake the urine will be concentrated and look dark yellow or amber.
   (B) This could indicate a urinary tract infection or a small amount of blood in the urine.
   (C) This could indicate blood in the urine due to a kidney problem or urinary tract infection.
   (D) This is the color of normal urine.

8. *(A) Fluid has mass and when it is retained, the person will gain weight.
   (B) Incontinence is related to the lack of bladder control, not the amount of fluid intake.
   (C) Extra fluid intake is flushed out through the kidneys, not through the intestines.
   (D) This would happen if the fluid intake were increased.

9. (A) A sign of constipation is hard, dry, formed stools, not tarry stools.
   *(B) Blood in the digestive system is acted on by the acids and enzymes, causing it to turn the stool black or tarry in color.
   (C) Diarrhea is usually related to food intolerances or intestinal infections, not tarry stools.
   (D) Gas in the intestines causes abdominal cramps and distention, not tarry stools.

10. *(A) An enema puts fluid into the large intestine; the pressure and irritation cause the colon to empty of stool.
    (B) An enema empties the intestine of stool; a urinary catheter (Foley catheter) drains the urinary bladder of urine.
    (C) An enema will not affect nausea and vomiting; nothing by mouth and medication can be used to limit nausea and vomiting.
    (D) A Harris drip (Harris flush) helps get rid of intestinal gas, not increase the passage of stool.

11. (A) Adequate fluid intake keeps the stool soft, which prevents constipation.
    *(B) People who are not active have decreased bowel activity (decreased peristalsis), which promotes constipation.
    (C) Bran is fiber that increases bowel activity and passage of stool.
    (D) People who get medication to promote passage of stool should not get constipated.

12. (A) Not the first step; the resident's usual voiding pattern must be identified before a plan can be developed.
    (B) Same as (A).
    *(C) What the resident usually does will determine how often the bedpan must be offered.
    (D) Not the first step; when retraining the bladder the resident may be encouraged to delay voiding.

13. (A) An unnecessary step if the resident cannot cooperate; this would be the first step after it is determined that the resident can cooperate.
     (B) Not effective if the resident cannot cooperate.
     *(C) This must be done first; unless the resident can cooperate, the rest of the steps will be useless.
     (D) Same as (B).

14. (A) This would be higher than the level of the bladder and could result in urine flowing back into the bladder.
     *(B) This allows urine to flow by gravity and prevents urine from flowing backward into the bladder.
     (C) Never clamp a Foley catheter; clamping can cause urine to back up into the bladder.
     (D) This would open what should be a closed system; closed systems prevent microorganisms from entering and causing infection.

15. (A) The collection bag would be above the level of the bladder; this could allow urine to flow backward into the bladder, which could cause infection.
     (B) Same as (A).
     (C) The urinary collection bag would become contaminated when placed on the floor.
     *(D) This would keep the urinary collection bag off the floor and below the level of the bladder, where it could drain by gravity.

16. *(A) The urinary catheter is too small and needs to be replaced by a larger-size catheter.
     (B) This addresses the need for skin care, but it does not solve the cause of the problem.
     (C) This will help keep the bed linen clean and dry, but it will not solve the cause of the problem.
     (D) A urinary catheter keeps the bladder empty; there should be no urge to void because of urine in the bladder.

17. (A) A urinary condom should cover the full length of the penis.
     *(B) The penis should be dry; wetting the penis would prevent the urinary condom device from staying on; also, moisture promotes the growth of microorganisms and causes skin breakdown.
     (C) This would keep pressure off the catheter and allow urine to flow into the drainage bag.
     (D) Keeping the drainage bag below the level of the bladder allows urine to flow toward the bag by gravity.

RESPIRATORY AND CIRCULATORY NEEDS

This section includes questions related to signs of abnormal respiratory functioning, the abdominal thrust, methods to improve circulation, and methods to improve respiration such as positioning and administering oxygen.

Questions

1. A nurse aide (NA) should know that a resident is not getting enough oxygen when the resident's fingernail beds are:
   (A) Pink.
   (B) Yellow.
   (C) Blue.
   (D) Beige.

2. Which of the following signs and symptoms of respiratory distress should the NA immediately report to the nurse?
   (A) Respirations of 14, regular rhythm
   (B) Respirations of 18, shallow breathing
   (C) Respirations of 20, regular rhythm
   (D) Respirations of 34, shallow breathing

3. A resident has a history of difficulty breathing because of chronic respiratory disease. Which of the following should be immediately reported to the nurse?
   (A) Refusing to lie down in bed
   (B) Wheezing sounds when breathing
   (C) Shortness of breath after walking
   (D) Bright red mucus from the mouth

4. Overweight (obese) residents often have the most trouble breathing when positioned:
   (A) Flat on their backs (supine position).
   (B) With the head of the bed raised (semi-Fowler's position).
   (C) With the head raised and knees gatched (contour position).
   (D) In a wheelchair (sitting position).

5. To increase both the respiratory and the circulatory functions of a resident in a coma, what is the MOST important thing the NA should do?
   (A) Massage the resident's bony areas.
   (B) Change the resident's position every two hours.
   (C) Explain to the resident how to cough.
   (D) Assist the resident with breathing exercises.

6. The doctor orders elastic stockings for Mrs. Henry. The NA should put the stockings on the resident:

    (A) When she is ready to go to bed at night.

    (B) In the afternoon when her feet swell.

    (C) When she complains that her feet hurt.

    (D) Before she gets out of bed in the morning.

7. The Fowler's position is used to relieve:

    (A) Difficult breathing.

    (B) Edema of the legs.

    (C) Pressure on the buttocks.

    (D) Flexion of the hips.

8. If a resident chokes on a piece of food and cannot speak, what should the NA do first?

    (A) Call the nurse immediately.

    (B) Begin cardiopulmonary resuscitation (CPR).

    (C) Pound three times on the resident's chest.

    (D) Perform the Heimlich maneuver.

9. Why are abdominal thrusts done in the Heimlich maneuver?

    (A) To pump the heart

    (B) To put pressure on the stomach

    (C) To push air out of the lungs

    (D) To produce a burp

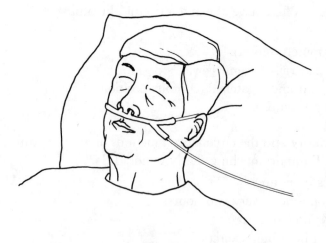

10. The tube pictured above is used to:

    (A) Administer oxygen.

    (B) Suction mucus.

    (C) Provide food.

    (D) Collect waste.

11. The resident is getting oxygen through a nasal cannula. Which of the following actions should not be done to prevent skin breakdown?

    (A) Adjust the cannula strap so it is comfortable.
    (B) Remove the cannula every two hours for 15 minutes.
    (C) Clean the nose and nose openings every shift.
    (D) Provide mouth care every two hours.

12. When a resident is placed on oxygen therapy, what is the first thing the NA should do?

    (A) Teach the resident not to smoke.
    (B) Move the resident to a private room.
    (C) Place a fire extinguisher in the room.
    (D) Position the resident flat in bed.

13. The resident is receiving oxygen through a face mask and complains that the elastic strap is too tight. The NA should:

    (A) Immediately tell the nurse.
    (B) Slightly loosen the elastic strap.
    (C) Gently remove the face mask.
    (D) Firmly explain that it has to stay that way.

Reasons for Answers

The asterisk (*) is in front of the correct answer.

1.   (A) This is an expected color of fingernail beds.
     (B) This could be due to jaundice or a fungus under the nail.
    *(C) A blue tinge to the fingernail beds, which are far from the heart, is a sign of a lack of oxygen.
     (D) Same as (A).

2.   (A) This is within normal limits for rate and characteristics of respirations.
     (B) Same as (A).
     (C) Same as (A).
    *(D) A respiratory rate of 34 is too fast; fast, shallow breathing means the person is having an oxygen problem.

3.   (A) This is common among people with chronic respiratory disease; keeping the head up helps breathing.
     (B) This is common with chronic respiratory disease; if it gets worse, then it should be reported.
     (C) Same as (B).
    *(D) This indicates bleeding in the lungs or breathing passages and should be immediately reported.

4. *(A) The weight of the chest and abdomen puts pressure on the diaphragm, which makes it hard to take a breath.
     (B) This helps breathing because the abdominal organs drop by gravity, which allows the chest to expand and the diaphragm to move down when breathing in.
     (C) Same as (B).
     (D) Same as (B).

5.   (A) This only helps skin circulation in the small area being massaged.
    *(B) This helps respirations by preventing fluid from collecting in the lung, which can cause infection; it helps circulation since activity increases circulation, and it relieves pressure.
     (C) Residents in a coma are unable to respond to directions.
     (D) Same as (A).

6.   (A) Elastic stockings are usually removed during sleep; blood flow back to the heart is adequate when the legs are level with the heart.
     (B) Elastic stockings should not be put on once there is extra fluid in the tissues because it could injure the tissues.
     (C) Elastic stockings should be applied before getting out of bed to prevent discomfort.
    *(D) Elastic stockings should be applied before fluid collects in the tissues; fluid collects in the tissues of the lower legs due to standing and sitting (dependent edema).

7. *(A) In the Fowler's position the abdominal organs drop down, which provides more space in the chest for the lungs to expand.

(B) Elevation of the legs reduces leg swelling (edema).

(C) In the Fowler's position the buttocks bear most of the weight of the body.

(D) A Fowler's position places the hips in flexion.

8. (A) There may not be enough time to find the nurse; an airway obstruction can rapidly lead to cardiac arrest.

(B) This may cause further obstruction by forcing the food lower into the breathing passages.

(C) Same as (B).

*(D) Abdominal thrusts push air out of the lungs, forcing out the food that is causing the obstruction.

9. (A) Pressing on the heart (compression) is used in cardiopulmonary resuscitation (CPR).

(B) Whatever is causing the obstruction is not caught in the esophagus, which leads to the stomach, but in the respiratory system.

*(C) When trapped air behind an obstruction is forced out, it pushes out what is causing the obstruction.

(D) Same as (B).

10. *(A) This is a nasal cannula, used to deliver oxygen from an oxygen tank or wall oxygen to the nose.

(B) A nasal cannula is pictured, not a suction tube to remove mucus.

(C) A nasal cannula is pictured, not a nasogastric tube, which goes into the nose, down the esophagus, and into the stomach to deliver food.

(D) A nasal cannula is pictured, not a urinary tube (Foley catheter), which goes into the urinary bladder, not the nose.

11. (A) If too tight the strap can cause pressure sores.

*(B) Oxygen should never be removed except to clean the nose and its openings quickly.

(C) This should be done every shift and whenever necessary to remove mucus and debris.

(D) This helps to limit the drying effect that oxygen has on the mucous membranes of the nose and mouth.

12. *(A) Residents receiving oxygen should be taught all safety rules related to oxygen therapy; oxygen supports fire.

(B) This is not necessary.

(C) Same as (B).

(D) People with breathing problems should be positioned in a semi- or high Fowler's position.

13. (A) This is not an emergency; the NA can adjust the elastic strap to make it more comfortable.

   *(B) The NA can adjust the elastic strap to make it more comfortable as long as the edges of the mask are still against the skin.

    (C) Unsafe; this would cut off the resident's oxygen supply.

    (D) The resident can receive oxygen and still be comfortable; the strap is too tight and needs to be slightly loosened.

BEHAVIORAL CHANGES AND PSYCHOSOCIAL PROBLEMS

The section includes questions on resident's rights and identifying and meeting resident's emotional, social, and spiritual needs.

Questions

1. An alert and oriented resident is having trouble remembering questions for the doctor. To help her overcome the problem of forgetting, what should the nurse aide (NA) do?
   (A) Remind her of the next doctor's visit.
   (B) Give her a pad and pencil.
   (C) Take her to and from the doctor's visit.
   (D) Post a calendar in her room.

2. Which of the following would NOT help to reduce a resident's confusion?
   (A) Maintain a set routine.
   (B) Orient to time, place, and person.
   (C) Play the radio louder than normal.
   (D) Give clear directions when giving care.

3. The resident is disoriented, has limited thinking ability, and is unable to make decisions because of damage to the brain. When caring for this resident, what should the NA do?
   (A) Give simple directions.
   (B) Offer her choices.
   (C) Say nothing.
   (D) Increase her activities.

4. A resident becomes easily confused. To meet his nutritional needs, what is the **best** thing the NA should do?
   (A) Feed him all his meals.
   (B) Set up the tray like a clock.
   (C) Encourage the intake of foods with vitamin A.
   (D) Offer him support throughout the meal.

5. Mrs. Corona talks a lot about her early life and tries to keep the NA from leaving the room. What should the NA do?
   (A) Explain to her that there are others who need care.
   (B) Tell her to look to the future and forget the past.
   (C) Set aside time to listen to her stories.
   (D) Sit her near a confused resident who will listen.

6. The resident is confused and does not understand what is happening around him. Which of the following forms of communication by the NA would *most* likely cause a good response?
   (A) Hugging
   (B) Directions
   (C) Talking
   (D) Pictures

7. A resident has not been eating or sleeping well and has lost all interest in activities of daily living. These behaviors indicate:
   (A) Anger
   (B) Depression
   (C) Denial
   (D) Acceptance

8. When the NA is giving Mr. Ford care, he sadly talks about how hard he was on his children when they were growing up. What is the BEST response by the NA?
   (A) ''Sounds like you were a tough Dad.''
   (B) Raise the eyebrows, but say nothing.
   (C) ''You feel you were hard on the children?''
   (D) ''How are they doing now?''

9. A dying resident says to the NA, ''I really don't want to go on living. When I get the chance I'm going to kill myself.'' What should the NA do?
   (A) Tell the nurse right away.
   (B) Watch the resident closely.
   (C) Share this with the evening NA.
   (D) Provide for confidentiality and tell no one.

10. A resident with cancer has pain that prevents him from doing even simple tasks for himself. Which of the following behaviors would show that he is depressed?
    (A) Holding the painful area with his hand
    (B) Showing sadness and loss of appetite
    (C) Hitting and biting care givers
    (D) Thinking his roommate wants to hurt him

11. Mrs. Drake is weak and unsteady on her feet. She insists on going to the bathroom by herself without calling for help. The NA recognizes this behavior as:
    (A) An inability to accept her limitations.
    (B) A desire to do something exciting.
    (C) An attempt to upset the staff.
    (D) A concern about not bothering others.

12. Mrs. Sear has poor vision and is afraid to leave her room because she may fall. What should the NA do?

    (A) Tell her not to be afraid.
    (B) Provide activities in her room.
    (C) Assist her to and from activities outside her room.
    (D) Let her use a wheelchair so she does not fall.

13. Mrs. Tiggs is hard of hearing and says that others are talking about her. What should the NA do?

    (A) Advise her to stay away from others.
    (B) Shout to her in a loud voice.
    (C) Tell her others are not talking about her.
    (D) Encourage her to attend activity programs.

14. Mrs. Spirit is paranoid and thinks that people are out to get her. When giving care, what is the **most** important thing the NA should do?

    (A) Explain everything that is to be done.
    (B) Always tell her how nice she looks.
    (C) Accept all the resident's behavior.
    (D) Tell her what she wants to hear.

15. Mrs. Pole is active in activities, has friends, and appears happy. When her son visits each week she cries, complains of pain, and tells him how unhappy she is. What should the NA do?

    (A) Tell the resident to stop upsetting the son.
    (B) Say nothing and stay out of it.
    (C) Tell the nurse so the nurse can deal with this problem.
    (D) Explain to the son that she only behaves this way when he visits.

16. Mr. Breeze is 99 years old. As his birthday gets closer he refuses to have a birthday party and gets upset whenever anyone mentions his age. The NA recognizes this behavior as:

    (A) Denial.
    (B) Guilt.
    (C) Loneliness.
    (D) Sadness.

17. Mrs. Rail is admitted to a nursing home. She begins to cry as her family leaves. Which of the following is the probable reason for her crying?

    (A) Anger
    (B) Anxiety
    (C) Guilt
    (D) Denial

18. A resident has a caring doctor and yet the resident complains that the doctor does not know what he is doing. She says he ignores her and is mean. The NA recognizes that the basis for this reaction is:

    (A) Regression.
    (B) Anxiety.
    (C) Denial.
    (D) Anger.

19. Mrs. Cox is grouchy, bossy and sometimes hits the NA. When giving her care, what should the NA do?

    (A) Include her in as many decisions as possible.
    (B) Avoid her when she is angry.
    (C) Explain that the staff is only trying to help her.
    (D) Stop her grouchy and abusive behavior.

20. Mrs. Gates has diabetes and is told that she will need an amputation of her leg. She says to the NA, "If they only remove my toes, I promise to watch my diet better." The NA recognizes that she is going through which of the following stages of grieving?

    (A) Denial—1st stage
    (B) Anger—2nd stage
    (C) Bargaining—3rd stage
    (D) Depression—4th stage

21. Mrs. Adams is grieving the recent death of her husband. She begins to cry. What should the NA do?

    (A) Look away when she cries.
    (B) Stay with her while she cries.
    (C) Encourage her to get involved in activities.
    (D) Suggest that she think about happy things.

22. Mr. Allen is angry because he can no longer do many things for himself. What should the NA do to make him feel less angry?

    (A) Tell him what he should do.
    (B) Assist him with all his care.
    (C) Encourage him to accept his dependence.
    (D) Give him choices about his care.

23. A resident is dying and is sad, withdrawn, and crying. What should the NA do?

    (A) Stay with the resident as much as possible.
    (B) Encourage the resident to bargain with God.
    (C) Provide a sunny environment.
    (D) Talk about things that are cheerful.

24. Mrs. Shor is terminally ill (dying). Which of the following is NOT an expected response when someone is grieving?
    (A) Talking about the illness
    (B) Getting angry at people
    (C) Feeling sad
    (D) Hearing voices

25. When giving care to dying residents, the NA should know the following fact about the stages of death and dying.
    (A) People will, in time, reach acceptance.
    (B) People can move back and forth between stages.
    (C) People should pass through the stages smoothly.
    (D) People must pass through the stages in order.

26. Mr. Stein has advanced lung cancer that is spreading fast, and he is coughing. While being given care, he says, "This cough is nothing. It's just a little cold. I'll be fine." How should the NA respond?
    (A) "It's not a cold, it's lung cancer."
    (B) "Tell me about this cough you have."
    (C) "Don't worry, the cough will go away."
    (D) "Let's talk about your lung cancer."

27. A dying (terminally ill) resident says to the NA, "My only fear is dying alone." What should the NA say?
    (A) "Don't worry. I'll be with you."
    (B) "You are afraid of dying alone?"
    (C) "Your family can stay with you."
    (D) "There is always someone here, just ring."

28. A resident had pain yesterday. Whom should the NA talk with to find out if he is in pain today?
    (A) The nurse
    (B) The resident
    (C) The doctor
    (D) The roommate

29. All of the following are emotional reactions to moderate pain except:
    (A) Moaning.
    (B) Increased heart rate.
    (C) Refusing to move.
    (D) Complaints of suffering.

Reasons for the answers

The asterisk (*) is in front of the correct answer.

1. (A) It is not the visits she forgets, but the questions she wants to ask the doctor.
   *(B) This promotes independence and is helpful to residents with memory loss.
   (C) The resident has no problem with mobility.
   (D) Same as (A).

2. (A) This reduces confusion because a routine is familiar and the person knows what to expect.
   (B) Reorientation helps to jog a person's memory.
   *(C) This may be necessary for a person with a hearing loss, but it does not help orient a confused resident; the increased noise could increase confusion.
   (D) A short, simple statement is the best way to send a message to a confused resident.

3. *(A) A simple message is easier to understand by mentally impaired residents.
   (B) This will only increase restlessness and agitation; she is unable to make decisions.
   (C) This will cause isolation and increase fear.
   (D) This could increase confusion and fear; simple routines keep the amount of stimuli low.

4. (A) Not necessary; this would encourage dependence.
   (B) While this would be helpful, it does not keep the resident focused on the task of eating.
   (C) Vitamin A will not improve his vision; a well-balanced diet is adequate.
   *(D) Encouragement keeps him focused on the task at hand.

5. (A) This cuts off communication and may make her feel less worthy or guilty.
   (B) Life review is healthy and can help reduce anxiety, guilt, etc.
   *(C) This will help meet needs for self-esteem and belonging.
   (D) This resident is alert and needs appropriate feedback; residents should not be expected to give care or meet the needs of other residents.

6. *(A) A hug is a simple form of communication that even the most mentally impaired person may understand.
   (B) This requires understanding a spoken message.
   (C) Same as (B).
   (D) This requires understanding a visual message.

7. (A) Acting out behaviors such as being loud or abusive are behaviors related to anger.

   *(B) When people are depressed they usually turn inward and do not interact with others or the environment.

   (C) This is when a person refuses to believe or accept facts.

   (D) This is the 5th stage of grieving/dying where a person accepts the situation and is at peace.

8. (A) This makes a value judgment or a conclusion about a person based on the NA's own values and should be avoided.

   (B) This nonverbal action shows surprise and lack of acceptance and should be avoided.

   *(C) This allows the resident to talk about his feelings, which may include guilt that was never resolved.

   (D) This takes the focus off the resident's feelings of guilt and should be avoided.

9. *(A) The resident's life is in danger, and the nurse responsible for the well-being of the resident must immediately know this information.

   (B) This would not alert the nurse responsible for the care of this resident.

   (C) Same as (B).

   (D) Telling the nurse would not break confidentiality because the nurse is part of the health team and should know this information.

10. (A) Not a sign of depression; this is self-splinting and is an attempt to lessen the pain.

    *(B) These are classic and common signs of depression.

    (C) This is a form of self-defense or anger, not depression.

    (D) This is paranoid behavior, not depression.

11. *(A) Refusing help is an attempt to convince herself that she is still able.

    (B) She is seeking independence, not excitement.

    (C) She is seeking independence, not trying to upset the staff.

    (D) While this could also be true, the main driving force behind this behavior is the need for independence.

12. (A) This denies her feelings and will not reduce her fear.

    (B) This will increase social isolation and should be avoided.

    *(C) This provides for physical safety, which should reduce fear.

    (D) Not necessary; mobility is not the problem, fear of falling is the problem.

13. (A) This increases social isolation and promotes depression.

    (B) Not necessary; speaking clearly, slowly, and directly in front of the resident should support communication.

    (C) This denies feelings and may be false reassurance; it also cuts off communication.

    *(D) This will reduce social isolation that occurs with hearing loss; getting to know others may reduce feelings of not being accepted.

14. *(A) The care giver must be honest and open for trust to develop within people, especially with people who are paranoid.
     (B) This may not always be true; trust cannot develop if people feel they are being humored.
     (C) Limits must be set on dangerous behavior; paranoid people can be so fearful that they can cause injury to themselves and others.
     (D) Trust is based on honesty; at times disagreements cannot be avoided; avoid supporting the paranoid thinking.

15. (A) This denies the resident's feelings, passes judgment, and cuts off communication.
     (B) This observation is important and should be shared with the nurse.
    *(C) The behavior is attempting to control the son and needs an experienced professional to help the resident and son gain insight to the reasons for the behavior.
     (D) This should be handled by the nurse, who is better prepared to deal with the situation.

16. *(A) This behavior is an effort to deny aging.
     (B) This is when a person regrets having done something or not having done something.
     (C) This is a fear of not receiving warmth and comfort from others (emotional isolation).
     (D) Once the person emotionally recognizes that he is aging, then he may become sad.

17. (A) Usually when people are angry, they are verbally or nonverbally hostile.
    *(B) Changes in life patterns can cause anxiety; crying is a common sign of anxiety.
     (C) Crying is not a common response to guilt; feeling sorry and avoidance are more common responses to guilt.
     (D) Crying is not a sign of denial; denial is a refusal to believe facts.

18. (A) Regression is returning to childlike behavior.
    *(B) Anxiety can cause a person to be fearful or angry with others, which may be undeserved; this is a coping response called displacement.
     (C) Denial is refusing to accept.
     (D) Although she appears angry with the doctor, anxiety, not anger, is the basis of her behavior.

19. *(A) This supports her need to be in control.
     (B) This ignores her needs and feelings; it isolates her further just when she needs human contact.
     (C) This confronts her dependence and is not supportive of her need to be in control.
     (D) It is all right for residents to express anger as long as it is done in socially acceptable ways.

20. (A) Denial is indicated by the statement, "Not me."
    (B) Anger is indicated by the statement, "Why me?"
    *(C) This is bargaining; it is an attempt to put off the amputation by making a deal; bargaining is indicated by the statement, "Yes me, but . . ."
    (D) Depression is indicated by the statement, "Yes me."

21. (A) Not necessary; this may be done by care givers to make themselves feel more comfortable.
    *(B) This provides emotional support and shows acceptance and concern.
    (C) This denies her feelings.
    (D) Same as (C).

22. (A) This will only point out his dependence and make him more angry.
    (B) Same as (A).
    (C) Same as (A).
    *(D) This puts him in control and supports independence.

23. *(A) The true impact of dying is being realized, and the person needs to express sorrow; quiet contact from staff members is needed.
    (B) Inappropriate; the resident is past the 3rd stage, bargaining, and is in the 4th stage, depression.
    (C) Inappropriate; in the 4th stage of grieving, depression, residents lose interest in their surroundings and become withdrawn and quiet.
    (D) This ignores the resident's feelings of sadness and cuts off communication.

24. (A) Talking about the illness is expected; it helps to impress on the mind that the illness is reality.
    (B) This is anger, the 2nd stage of grieving; this acting out of angry feelings is often directed at family or staff members.
    (C) This is depression, the 4th stage of grieving; this is a sense of sadness.
    *(D) This is hallucinating and is not a stage in the grieving process.

25. (A) Some people never reach the 5th stage of acceptance.
    *(B) Grieving is not always a smooth passage from one stage to the next; people can move back and forth between stages, which can be frightening and confusing.
    (C) Incorrect; grieving is not always a smooth passage from one stage to the next.
    (D) Incorrect; people may move back and forth between stages.

26. (A) The resident is in the stage of denial and is not ready to face that he is dying; never take away a person's means of coping; this would cut off communication.
    *(B) This gives him the chance to talk about the "cough" that is bothering him; allows him to face the diagnosis when he is ready.
    (C) False reassurance; he is terminally ill and he will not get better.
    (D) Same as (A).

27. (A) This is false reassurance; an employee cannot be there 24 hours a day.
   *(B) This lets the resident talk more about his feelings.
   (C) The family may not be able or willing to stay; also, it ignores the resident's feelings.
   (D) This is false reassurance; the resident may not be able to ring; it does not address the fear.

28. (A) The nurse may know, but the information may not be as up to date as talking with the resident.
   *(B) The resident is the best source because he is the one feeling the pain; also, the information will be up to date.
   (C) The doctor is usually not at the nursing home all the time and is not always aware of the daily comfort needs of a resident.
   (D) Residents are not responsible for other residents.

29. (A) Moaning is an emotional reaction a person can control (voluntary); it is a behavior, not a physical response.
   *(B) An increased heart rate is not something most people can control; it is a physical attempt by the body to prepare for an emergency or threat.
   (C) This is an attempt to protect the painful area, a conscious behavior of the resident.
   (D) Talking about suffering is an emotional response to pain.

TEST DRILL 1

BLACKEN THE LETTER BOX BELOW WHICH MATCHES EACH LETTER OF YOUR NAME.

YOUR LAST NAME   YOUR FIRST NAME   MI

TEACHER ONLY: STUDENT ABSENT FOR PART: I II III IV

SEMESTER FALL SPRING

A B

STUDENT NUMBER

BIRTH DATE MO YEAR

SEX

GRADE

FORM OF THIS TEST IS: A 1   B 2   C 3   D 4

JAN FEB MAR APR MAY JUN JUL AUG SEP OCT NOV DEC

SCHOOL

CITY

GRADE

TEST

INSTRUCTOR

	A B C D E		A B C D E		A B C D E		A B C D E		A B C D E		A B C D E		A B C D E		A B C D E
1		6		11		16		21		26		31		36	
2		7		12		17		22		27		32		37	
3		8		13		18		23		28		33		38	
4		9		14		19		24		29		34		39	
5		10		15		20		25		30		35		40	
41		46		51		56		61		66		71		76	
42		47		52		57		62		67		72		77	
43		48		53		58		63		68		73		78	
44		49		54		59		64		69		74		79	
45		50		55		60		65		70		75		80	
81		86		91		96		101		106		111		116	
82		87		92		97		102		107		112		117	
83		88		93		98		103		108		113		118	
84		89		94		99		104		109		114		119	
85		90		95		100		105		110		115		120	
121		126		131		136		141		146		151		156	
122		127		132		137		142		147		152		157	
123		128		133		138		143		148		153		158	
124		129		134		139		144		149		154		159	
125		130		135		140		145		150		155		160	

TEST DRILL 2